Rotator Cuff Surgery

Guest Editor

STEPHEN F. BROCKMEIER, MD

CLINICS IN
SPORTS MEDICINE

www.sportsmed.theclinics.com

Consulting Editor
MARK D. MILLER, MD

October 2012 • Volume 31 • Number 4

SAUNDERS an imprint of ELSEVIER, Inc.

W.B. SAUNDERS COMPANY
A Division of Elsevier Inc.

1600 John F. Kennedy Blvd. ● Suite 1800 ● Philadelphia, Pennsylvania 19103

http://www.theclinics.com

CLINICS IN SPORTS MEDICINE Volume 31, Number 4
October 2012 ISSN 0278-5919, ISBN-13: 978-1-4557-4948-5

Editor: David Parsons

Clinics in Sports Medicine (ISSN 0278-5919) is published quarterly by Elsevier Inc., 360 Park Avenue South, New York, NY 10010-1710. Months of issue are January, April, July, and October. Business and Editorial Offices: 1600 John F. Kennedy Blvd., Ste. 1800, Philadelphia, PA 19103-2899. Customer Service Office: 3251 Riverport Lane, Maryland Heights, MO 63043. Periodicals postage paid at New York, NY and additional mailing offices. Subscription prices are $324.00 per year (US individuals), $503.00 per year (US institutions), $160.00 per year (US students), $367.00 per year (Canadian individuals), $608.00 per year (Canadian institutions), $223.00 (Canadian students), $446.00 per year (foreign individuals), $608.00 per year (foreign institutions), and $223.00 per year (foreign students). Foreign air speed delivery is included in all *Clinics* subscription prices. All prices are subject to change without notice. **POSTMASTER:** Send address changes to *Clinics in Sports Medicine*, Elsevier Health Sciences Division, Subscription Customer Service, 3251 Riverport Lane, Maryland Heights, MO 63043. Customer Service (orders, claims, online, change of address): Elsevier Health Sciences Division, Subscription Customer Service, 3251 Riverport Lane, Maryland Heights, MO 63043. Tel: 1-800-654-2452 (U.S. and Canada); 314-447-8871 (outside U.S. and Canada). Fax: 314-447-8029. E-mail: journals customerservice-usa@elsevier.com (for print support); journalsonlinesupport-usa@elsevier.com (for online support).

Reprints. For copies of 100 or more of articles in this publication, please contact the Commercial Reprints Department, Elsevier Inc., 360 Park Avenue South, New York, NY 10010-1710. Tel.: 212-633-3812; Fax: 212-462-1935; E-mail: reprints@elsevier.com.

Clinics in Sports Medicine is covered in *MEDLINE/PubMed (Index Medicus) Current Contents/Clinical Medicine, Excerpta Medica,* and *ISI/Biomed.*

Printed and bound by CPI Group (UK) Ltd, Croydon, CR0 4YY

Transferred to digital print 2012

Contributors

CONSULTING EDITOR

MARK D. MILLER, MD
S. Ward Casscells Professor of Orthopaedic Surgery head, Division of Sports Medicine, University of Virginia; Team Physician, James Madison University, Miller Review Course, Charlottesville, Virginia

GUEST EDITOR

STEPHEN F. BROCKMEIER, MD
Sports Medicine & Shoulder Surgery, Assistant Professor, Department of Orthopaedic Surgery, University of Virginia, Charlottesville, Virginia

AUTHORS

ALEXANDER W. ALEEM, MD
Department of Orthopaedic Surgery, Washington University School of Medicine, Chesterfield, Missouri

MARK W. ANDERSON, MD
Professor, Radiology and Orthopaedic Surgery; Chief, Division of Musculoskeletal Imaging, The University of Virginia Health Sciences Center, Charlottesville, Virginia

MICHAEL E. ANGELINE, MD
Fellow Sports Medicine and Shoulder Surgery, Department of Orthopaedic Surgery; Sports Medicine and Shoulder Surgery Service, Hospital for Special Surgery, New York, New York

CRIS D. BARNTHOUSE, MD
Orthopaedic and Sports Medicine Clinic of Kansas City, Leawood, Kansas

CHRISTOPHER BRENNAN, MD
Clinical Instructor, Department of Radiology, The University of Virginia Health Sciences Center, Charlottesville, Virginia

STEPHEN F. BROCKMEIER, MD
Sports Medicine & Shoulder Surgery, Assistant Professor, Department of Orthopaedic Surgery, University of Virginia, Charlottesville, Virginia

ROBERT H. BROPHY, MD
Assistant Professor, Division of Sports Medicine, Department of Orthopaedic Surgery, Washington University School of Medicine, Chesterfield, Missouri

RUTH A. DELANEY, MB BCh, BAO, MRCS
Resident, Harvard Combined Orthopaedic Residency Program, Massachusetts General Hospital, Boston, Massachusetts

KOSTAS J. ECONOMOPOULOS, MD
Sports Medicine Fellow, Department of Orthopaedic Surgery, University of Virginia, Charlottesville, Virginia

SETH C. GAMRADT, MD
Department of Orthopaedic Surgery, David Geffen School of Medicine at UCLA, Los Angeles, California

JAY D. KEENER, MD
Assistant Professor, Shoulder and Elbow Service, Department of Orthopaedic Surgery, Washington University, St Louis, Missouri

ALBERT LIN, MD
Fellow, Harvard Shoulder Service, Massachusetts General Hospital, Boston, Massachusetts

AMIT MITTAL, MD
Clinical Instructor, Department of Radiology, The University of Virginia Health Sciences Center, Charlottesville, Virginia

SCOTT R. MONTGOMERY, MD
Department of Orthopaedic Surgery, David Geffen School of Medicine at UCLA, Los Angeles, California

ANAND M. MURTHI, MD
Department of Orthopaedic Surgery, Union Memorial Hospital, Baltimore, Maryland

FRANK A. PETRIGLIANO, MD
Department of Orthopaedic Surgery, David Geffen School of Medicine at UCLA, Los Angeles, California

JOSE RAMIREZ, MA
Columbia College of Physicians and Surgeons, New York, New York

MIGUEL A. RAMIREZ, MD
Department of Orthopaedic Surgery, Union Memorial Hospital, Baltimore, Maryland

SCOTT A. RODEO, MD
Attending Orthopaedic Surgeon, Department of Orthopaedic Surgery; Co-Chief, Sports Medicine and Shoulder Surgery Service, Hospital for Special Surgery, New York, New York

ANDREW R. SCOTT, MD
Orthopaedic and Sports Medicine Clinic of Kansas City, Leawood, Kansas

ROBERT Z. TASHJIAN, MD
Associate Professor, Shoulder and Elbow Surgery, Department of Orthopaedics, University of Utah School of Medicine, Salt Lake City, Utah

JAMES E. VOOS, MD
Orthopaedic and Sports Medicine Clinic of Kansas City, Leawood, Kansas

JON J.P. WARNER, MD
Chief, Harvard Shoulder Service; Professor of Orthopaedics, Harvard Medical School, Massachusetts General Hospital, Boston, Massachusetts

Contents

Rotator cuff disease is the most common shoulder disorder treated by orthopedic surgeons. Little information exits regarding its prevalence and natural history. The prevalence of rotator cuff tearing increases with age as well as several other factors including smoking and family history. Knowledge regarding the natural history of nonoperatively treated tears as well as the healing potential after repair can be used to aid in refining surgical and nonsurgical indications for the treatment rotator cuff tears. An algorithmic approach to the treatment of rotator cuff tears is reviewed.

The rotator cuff is a complex network of interwoven tendons that plays a key role in glenohumeral movement and stability. Cuff abnormality is a common source of shoulder pain, but the clinical presentation is often nonspecific and, as a result, diagnostic imaging, especially magnetic resonance imaging, plays a key role in evaluating these patients. This article reviews imaging modalities available for evaluating the cuff, normal cuff anatomy, and common pathologic conditions that affect it.

Rotator cuff repairs have evolved from open to arthroscopic techniques. The fundamentals of recognizing rotator cuff tear patterns, tissue mobilization, footprint restoration, and stable repair construct remain largely unchanged. Recent clinical studies have raised concern regarding high retear rate for rotator cuff repairs, despite good clinical outcomes, with single-row repair techniques. As a result, double-row and transosseous-equivalent techniques have been developed. Biomechanical data favor these newer techniques whereas clinical data have not definitively concluded which technique is superior. The most up-to-date arthroscopic rotator cuff repair techniques are presented for partial-thickness and full-thickness rotator cuff tears.

Surgical repair of rotator cuff tears is a relatively common orthopedic procedure. Although the procedure is clinically successful, the repair site frequently has incomplete healing and gap formation, owing to a fibrovascular scar—mediated healing response at the tendon-bone interface. By augmenting the repair site with biological agents, the ultimate goal is to stimulate a regenerative healing pathway. Challenges remain, however, regarding the ideal factor(s), timing, and vehicle of delivery.

Rotator cuff tears are a common clinical problem that increases with age from an incidence of 4% in those aged 40 to 60 years to more than 54% in those older than 60 years. The purpose of this article is to review the current evidence regarding outcomes of surgical techniques in rotator cuff surgery. Future research should be aimed at identifying whether and in whom rotator cuff healing is appropriate to better identify surgical candidates as well as to determine the best surgical repair strategy.

Rotator cuff tears in overhead athletes can take on several different forms. Identification of symptomatic rotator cuff disease can be challenging in the overhead athlete as abnormalities of the rotator cuff can be seen commonly in asymptomatic throwers and rotator cuff pathologic conditions often occur in conjunction with other injuries. Partial-thickness tears treated with arthroscopic debridement and management of concomitant pathologic conditions appear to have fairly good outcomes in the literature with most athletes able to return to activity at their preinjury level. Full-thickness tears, however, have fared much more poorly in the overhead athlete with largely dismal outcomes after surgical repair.

Rotator cuff repair is performed commonly to address pain and shoulder dysfunction after a rotator cuff tear. Recurrent or persistent tears are common after rotator cuff repair. The causes of failed rotator cuff surgery include biologic factors, technical errors, and traumatic failure. A thorough history, physical examination, and appropriate imaging are required to determine if a patient is an appropriate candidate for revision rotator cuff repair. Ideal candidates for revision rotator cuff repair are younger, have minimal muscle atrophy, minimal tendon retraction, preoperative forward elevation of greater than 90°, a functioning deltoid, and no evidence of cuff tear arthropathy.

Rotator cuff repair is one of the most common procedures performed in the shoulder. Predictable pain relief and functional improvements are seen across all age groups. However, anatomic healing of the surgically repaired tendon is not as consistent and has varied widely in the literature.

The purpose of this article is to review the appropriate evaluation and management of patients with a failed rotator cuff repair, with specific emphasis on identifying proper surgical candidates for revision rotator cuff repair. This article also reviews the relevant surgical techniques, appropriate rehabilitation, and expected outcomes of revision rotator cuff repair surgery.

Massive, irreparable rotator cuff tears remain a clinical challenge. In low-demand patients, debridement of the tear may relieve pain. Partial repair using the technique of margin convergence decreases the size of the tear gap and reduces strain. Biceps tenotomy or tenodesis has a role in providing pain relief in massive rotator cuff tears. Tendon transfers offer good results in patients with massive, irreparable rotator cuff tears. The treatment modality specifically chosen for the massive, irreparable rotator cuff tear must be tailored to the individual patient, their needs and expectations, and their ability to comply with intensive rehabilitation.

Reverse shoulder arthroplasty (RSA) was pioneered by Grammont in the 1980s as a potential treatment for cuff tear arthropathy and irreparable cuff tears. RSA was designed to use the deltoid as the primary elevator of the shoulder, negating the need for the rotator cuff. Early short-term results show improvements in pain and function scores for both cuff tear arthropathy and irreparable cuff tears. Long-term studies are still needed to evaluate the long-term benefits of these devices in this patient population.

CLINICS IN SPORTS MEDICINE

Foreword

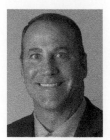

Mark D. Miller, MD
Guest Editor

When we realized how difficult it was to manage massive rotator cuff tears and rotator cuff arthropathy in our sports medicine practice at the University of Virginia, we recognized that we needed some help. That help materialized with the addition of the guest editor for this edition of *Clinics in Sports Management*, Dr Stephen Brockmeier. Because of his demonstrated expertise in this area since his matriculation to University of Virginia, I thought that it would be appropriate for him to develop a treatise on rotator cuff disease. I like to tell medical students and residents that rotator cuff disease is a continuum, beginning with partial cuff tears and progressing to massive, irreparable tears, and ultimately, rotator cuff arthropathy. This issue reinforces this concept and brings us all up to date on rotator cuff disease.

The edition begins with epidemiology, provides imaging updates, and then focuses on techniques and outcomes. The "advanced" articles include revision, massive, and irreparable tears and round out a comprehensive and complete discussion of rotator cuff problems. Congratulations to Dr Brockmeier for putting together a great issue, and best wishes to all of you as you take on these challenging cases!

Mark D. Miller, MD
S. Ward Casscells Professor of Orthopaedic Surgery
Head, Division of Sports Medicine
University of Virginia
Team Physician, James Madison University
Miller Review Course
400 Ray C. Hunt Drive, Suite 330
Charlottesville, VA 22908-0159, USA

E-mail address:
MDM3P@hscmail.mcc.virginia.edu

Clin Sports Med 31 (2012) ix
http://dx.doi.org/10.1016/j.csm.2012.08.001
0278-5919/12/$ – see front matter © 2012 Elsevier Inc. All rights reserved.

Preface

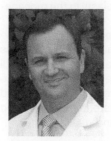

Stephen Brockmeier, MD
Guest Editor

The management of disorders of the rotator cuff continues to be an area of intense academic and clinical interest and controversy in the sports medicine world. From the overhead athlete to the elderly population, the spectrum of disease affects patients of all ages and all walks of life. Recent research has led to a better understanding of the etiology and natural history of rotator cuff disease, while improved surgical techniques have provided for an evolution in treatment. This issue of *Clinics in Sports Medicine* is dedicated to all things rotator cuff, with an emphasis on current areas of controversy, evolving management trends, and future paths of research and investigation.

To tackle this enormous topic, we have assembled a distinguished group of authors who each bring their unique level of experience and insight. The first article sets the stage for the entire issue, by presenting the current evidence on the epidemiology and natural history of rotator cuff disease. In this article, Dr Robert Tashjian from the University of Utah not only systematically reviews the evidence but also presents a thoughtful and logical treatment algorithm for management of rotator cuff tears. This is followed by an excellent review by Dr Mark Anderson and his coauthors from the University of Virginia detailing the imaging evaluation of the rotator cuff. Next, Dr James Voos provides a summary of the techniques of arthroscopic rotator cuff repair in 2012.

In the fourth article, Dr Michael Angeline and Dr Scott Rodeo from the Hospital for Special Surgery discuss the current status of biologics in the management of rotator cuff tears. This article is a highlight, providing not only the current level of evidence but what the future may hold in this area. Next, Drs Aleem and Brophy from Washington University review rotator cuff disease from an evidence-based medicine perspective. A review of the management of rotator cuff disorders in the overhead athlete follows with an emphasis on the unique features in this challenging subset of patients. Next, Drs Montgomery, Petrigliano, and Gamradt from UCLA detail the approach to the patient with a failed previous rotator cuff procedure. Dr Jay Keener then augments this with a discussion of revision rotator cuff surgery, highlighting the indications, evaluation, and management options in this setting.

The final 2 articles present potential salvage options in the setting of a massive and irreparable rotator cuff tear. Dr John JP Warner and his associates from Harvard tackle

Clin Sports Med 31 (2012) xi–xii
http://dx.doi.org/10.1016/j.csm.2012.08.002
0278-5919/12/$ – see front matter © 2012 Elsevier Inc. All rights reserved.

sportsmed.theclinics.com

a particularly difficult topic as they review nonarthroplasty options such as debridement, biceps surgery, suprascapular neurolysis, and tendon transfer. Finally, Dr Anand Murthi and coauthors discuss the role of reverse shoulder arthroplasty in the management of irreparable rotator cuff tears or rotator cuff arthropathy.

I would like to thank the editorial staff of *Clinics in Sport Management* for the privilege of overseeing the creation of this issue. I hope that you find the issue to be as fascinating and thought-provoking as I do. Most importantly, I am sincerely grateful to all of the contributing authors for taking the time to present their work and educate us all on this unique topic. These individuals are all on the cutting edge of this area and their contributions have helped to shape our understanding of rotator cuff disease and improve our ability to treat patients and improve their function and quality of life.

Stephen Brockmeier, MD
Sports Medicine & Shoulder Surgery
Assistant Professor
Department of Orthopaedic Surgery
University of Virginia

E-mail address:
sfb2e@virginia.edu

Epidemiology, Natural History, and Indications for Treatment of Rotator Cuff Tears

Robert Z. Tashjian, MD*

KEYWORDS

- Rotator cuff • Natural history • Tendon healing • Indications

KEY POINTS

- The etiology of rotator cuff tearing is multifactorial and likely a combination of age-related degenerative changes and microtrauma/macrotrauma. Smoking, hypercholesterolemia, and family history have been shown to predispose individuals to rotator cuff tearing.
- Full-thickness rotator cuff tears are present in approximately 25% of individuals in their 60s and 50% of individuals in their 80s.
- Asymptomatic full-thickness rotator cuff tears are common, increase in incidence with aging, and are present in approximately 50% of patients over age 65 with a contralateral symptomatic full-thickness tear; 50% of asymptomatic full-thickness tears develop symptoms in approximately 2 to 3 years and 50% of those developing symptoms progress in tear size. Larger asymptomatic tears are more likely to develop symptoms over time.
- Symptomatic full-thickness tears progress in tear size in approximately 50% of cases at an average of 2 years. Tear size progression is correlated with increasing symptoms. Small (<1–1.5 cm) full-thickness tears have a slower risk of tear size progression (25% at 2 years) compared with larger full-thickness tears.
- Partial-thickness symptomatic and asymptomatic tears progress in tear size at a slower rate than full-thickness tears and tear progression is associated with worsening pain.
- Early surgical repair can be considered for acute tears in any age group and in chronic, reparable tears in young patients (<65 years old) of substantial size (>1 cm) without significant chronic muscle changes.
- Initial nonoperative treatment should be considered in all patients with tendonitis, partial-thickness tears, small (<1–1.5 cm) full-thickness tears, all chronic tears in an older age group (>65 or 70 years), and all large irreparable tears with chronic, irreversible muscle changes.

Disclosures: Conflict of interest—none.
Funding source—Department of Orthopaedics, University of Utah, Veterans Administration Merit Review Grant.
Shoulder and Elbow Surgery, Department of Orthopaedics, University of Utah School of Medicine, Salt Lake City, UT, USA
* University of Utah Orthopaedic Center, 590 Wakara Way, Salt Lake City, UT 84108.
E-mail address: Robert.Tashjian@hsc.utah.edu

INTRODUCTION

Rotator cuff disorders are the most common cause of disability related to the shoulder.[1] Despite a large amount of literature on the management of rotator cuff tears, surgical indications remain controversial and are not standardized.[2] Potential reasons for this lack of consistent management of rotator cuff tears are the significant variability of clinical manifestations and a lack of information regarding the natural history of symptomatic tears.[3,4] Limited natural history information is likely due to many tears being surgically treated after the development of symptoms. By attempting to understand the natural history of rotator cuff tears, significant insight can be gained into the etiology of the disease process as well as an understanding of when early surgical intervention should be considered versus conservative care to limit irreversible rotator cuff changes.

In order to thoroughly define the indications for treatment of rotator cuff tears, the risks and benefits of both operative and nonoperative treatment must be fully examined. Although much attention has been focused on the relative risks and benefits of surgical intervention, the risks of nonoperative treatment are just as important when considering options. The basis for an organized approach to treating rotator cuff tears is grounded in the risk for chronic rotator cuff changes associated with nonoperative treatment, the potential for healing of partial-thickness and full-thickness tears, the reparability of tears, and the prognostic factors associated with functional outcomes after treatment. This article reviews the current data regarding the prevalence of rotator cuff tearing, the natural history of asymptomatic and symptomatic rotator cuff tears, the potential for healing after rotator cuff repair, and the indications for and timing of operative and nonoperative treatment of rotator cuff tears.

EPIDEMIOLOGY
Prevalence

Several investigators have attempted to estimate the prevalence of partial-thickness and full-thickness rotator cuff tears using both cadaver investigations and various imaging techniques in asymptomatic and symptomatic individuals. Cadaver and autopsy dissections have revealed a prevalence of rotator cuff tendon defects ranging from 5% to almost 40%.[5,6] Neer[6] reported that full-thickness tears occurred less than 5% of the time in more than 500 cadaveric specimens, whereas Lehman and colleagues[7] found full-thickness tears 17% of the time in 235 cadavers. The prevalence of full-thickness tears was 6% in specimens less than 60 years old as opposed to 30% in those older than 60.[7] Yamanaka and Fukada[8] reported a prevalence of supraspinatus full-thickness and partial-thickness tears of 7% and 13%, respectively, in a series of 249 cadavers. Partial-thickness tears were further grouped as bursal sided (2.4%), intratendinous (7.2%), and articular sided (3.6%).

Several investigators have evaluated shoulders in asymptomatic individuals with MRI and ultrasound in an attempt to determine the likelihood of rotator cuff tearing. Sher and colleagues[9] found the overall prevalence of tears in asymptomatic individuals to be 34% by MRI: 15% full thickness and 20% partial thickness. In patients older than 60 years of age, full-thickness and partial-thickness tears were found in 28% and 26% of individuals, respectively. In patients between 40 and 60 years of age, full-thickness and partial-thickness tears were found in 4% and 24% of individuals, respectively. Finally, no individuals less than 40 years old had a full-thickness tear, and 4% had partial-thickness tears. Tempelhof and colleagues[10] found, using ultrasound. an overall prevalence of full-thickness rotator cuff tears in asymptomatic individuals to be 23%, with 51% of individuals over age 80 having tears.

The major problem with the imaging studies previously described is that they evaluated only asymptomatic individuals. Yamaguchi and colleagues[11] evaluated patients presenting with unilateral shoulder pain with bilateral shoulder ultrasounds. They determined that cuff tearing increased incrementally with age. The average age of patients with bilateral intact cuffs was 48.7, a unilateral cuff tear was 58.7, and bilateral cuff tear was 67.8. If patients had a symptomatic rotator cuff tear, there was a 35% chance of a cuff tear on the opposite side, which increased to 50% if the patient was 66 years of age or older.

Yamamoto and colleagues[12] recently published a population-based study evaluating the prevalence of rotator cuff tearing in both symptomatic and asymptomatic individuals using ultrasound. Rotator cuff tears were present in 20.7% of individuals from a population of 683 patients; 36% of subjects with symptoms had a cuff tear whereas only 16.9% without symptoms had a cuff tear. Cuff tearing was associated with increasing age with 25.6% of individuals in their 60s having a tear, which increased up to 50% of individuals in their 80s. Increasing age, a history of trauma, and hand dominance were risk factors associated with tearing. These studies support the theory that rotator cuff tearing occurs, to some extent, as a normal degenerative process, which increases with aging, yet trauma, either microtrauma or macrotrauma, may also play a role in cuff tear development.

Risk Factors

Several patient-related risk factors have been identified predisposing individuals to the development of rotator cuff tears. Increasing patient age is probably the most important as the prevalence data suggest. Several other risk factors have been identified, including smoking, hypercholesterolemia, and family history. Each of these may play an additive role to the underlying influence of age-related degeneration in the development of rotator cuff disease.

Smoking

Limited blood supply to the critical portion of the rotator cuff has been described as potentially contributing to the development of rotator cuff tears.[13] Nicotine is a potent vasoconstrictor and decreases the delivery of oxygen to tissues.[14] Lower oxygen in the critical zone (hypovascular zone of the supraspinatus and infraspinatus tendons approximately 15 mm from their insertions) of the rotator cuff may lead to an increased risk for tearing.[15] Smoking has not only been shown to increase the risk for rotator cuff tearing but also has been associated with a predisposition for increased tear size, limited healing ability after repair, and poorer clinical outcomes after surgical repair.[16–19]

Baumgarten and colleagues[16] evaluated 586 consecutive patients presenting with shoulder pain with a questionnaire. A history of smoking (61.9% vs 48.3%), smoking within the previous 10 years (35.2% vs 30.1%), mean duration of smoking (23.4 vs 20.2 years), mean packs per day of smoking (1.25 vs 1.10 packs per day), and mean pack-years of smoking (30.1 vs 22.0) correlated with an increased risk for the presence of a rotator cuff tear. After age-adjustment through stratification, a history of smoking was still more prevalent in the rotator cuff tear group compared with the no-tear group.

Recently, Carbone and colleagues[17] evaluated the effects of smoking on tear size; 408 patients undergoing arthroscopic rotator cuff repair were included in the study. The investigators determined that the frequency of smokers was lower in patients with a small full-thickness tear (23.2%) versus a larger full-thickness tear (34.8%) ($P = .033$). Also, total number of cigarettes and number of daily cigarettes was significantly higher in patients with a larger tear as opposed to a small full-thickness tear ($P = .032$ and $P = .04$, respectively) after adjusting for age. Consequently, smoking seems to be an independent risk factor for the both the development of rotator cuff tears as well as increasing tear size.

Hypercholesterolemia

Deposition of cholesterol by-products has been implicated in increasing the risk for tendon rupture. Hypercholesterolemia has been evaluated in a mouse model and was shown to decrease the elastic modulus of an intact patellar tendon suggesting a detrimental effect of hypercholesterolemia on baseline tendon biomechanical properties.[20] Abboud and Kim[21] measured serum lipid profiles in 80 patients presenting with full-thickness rotator cuff tears and compared them to 80 controls with shoulder pain but a normal rotator cuff as confirmed by MRI. Total cholesterol, triglycerides, and low-density lipoprotein cholesterol concentrations of patients with rotator cuff tears were all significantly higher than levels in the control group; 64% of patients with a tear had an elevated serum cholesterol (total cholesterol greater than 240 mg/dL) compared with 28% in the control group. Consequently, hypercholesterolemia may have an additive role in the development of rotator cuff tearing.

Genetics

Familial predisposition has been suggested to increase the risk for the development of rotator cuff tearing. Harvie and colleagues[22] performed a sibling study where 129 siblings were retrospectively evaluated in a cohort of 205 patients diagnosed as having full-thickness rotator cuff tears by ultrasound. Using the spouses of the patients as a control group, the relative risk of full-thickness tears in siblings compared with controls was 2.42. Evaluation of the same population 5 years later showed that siblings were more likely to have had a progression of tear size (62.9% in siblings vs 22.1% in controls).[23] Drawbacks of the Harvie and colleagues[22] and the Gwilym and colleagues[23] studies included small sample sizes and a review of only close (first-degree) relatives. Tashjian and colleagues[24] performed an analysis to determine the genetic predisposition for rotator cuff tearing using a large population database. In a group of 3091 patients, the relative risk of rotator cuff disease in the relatives of patients diagnosed with cuff disease before age 40 years was significantly elevated for both second-degree and third-degree relatives. The observation of significantly elevated relative risks to both close and distant relatives strongly supports a heritable predisposition to rotator cuff disease. Further research is required to determine exactly what genetic variants predispose individuals to tearing.

NATURAL HISTORY OF ROTATOR CUFF DISEASE
Asymptomatic Full-Thickness Tears

The study of asymptomatic rotator cuff tears provides important information, including knowledge regarding the clinical manifestation of rotator cuff tears and the potential treatment options for symptomatic cuff tears that become asymptomatic. As discussed previously, a high percentage of individuals have asymptomatic rotator cuff tears. A significant number of these patients are at risk for the development of symptoms over time. Yamaguchi and colleagues[4] evaluated patients with symptomatic rotator cuff tears and a contralateral asymptomatic tear: 51% of the patients with a previously asymptomatic tear developed symptoms over an average of 2.8 years; 50% of the newly symptomatic tears progressed in size whereas only 20% of the tears that remained asymptomatic progressed in size. There was no evidence of tendon healing or decrease in tear size. These data suggest that the rotator cuff tendon has a limited ability to heal itself if left unrepaired. More importantly, there is a significant risk for tear progression, which is correlated with the development of symptoms.

Recently, Mall and Yamaguchi have reported on cohort patients with asymptomatic rotator cuff tears who became symptomatic and compared them to a matched group who remained asymptomatic.[25] They compared 34 patients who became symptomatic to 35 patients who remained asymptomatic. The cuff tears that became symptomatic developed symptoms approximately 2 years after the initial evaluation. In general, cuff tears in the symptom development group were significantly larger than those in the group that remained asymptomatic at their initial evaluation (P<.01). Also, tear enlargement was more common in the group that became symptomatic (23%) compared with those who remained asymptomatic (4%). Conclusions from this data are that larger tears are more likely to develop symptoms and that development of pain correlates with tear enlargement. Consequently, development of pain in asymptomatic tears should alert surgeons to evaluate the shoulder with an imaging study to evaluate tear enlargement.

Aside from progression in size, it is unclear what determines the clinical manifestation of a rotator cuff tear and why some tears become symptomatic. Burkhart[26] proposed the theory that normal glenohumeral kinematics can be preserved in the setting of a rotator cuff tear as long as the cuff's force couples are maintained. Tear size is less important than tear location in terms of force couple and kinematic preservation. Abnormal glenohumeral kinematics may be a precipitating factor for symptom development. Yamaguchi and colleagues[27] performed kinematic evaluations on asymptomatic patients with and without rotator cuff tears and symptomatic patients with tears and found abnormal kinematics in patients with tears. Both asymptomatic and symptomatic cuff tear patients demonstrated superior migration of the humeral head compared with controls. Keener and colleagues[28] followed-up this study to determine the effect of tear size and pain on kinematics. They also determined that migration occurred in both asymptomatic and symptomatic tears although migration was greater in the symptomatic tears (P = .03). The most important factor regarding migration was overall tear size (P = .01). These data suggest that abnormal glenohumeral kinematic function cannot independently explain the presence of symptoms and altered kinematics is probably most influenced by tear size.

Finally, differential muscle activation has been examined as a potential source of symptom development in rotator cuff tears. Kelly and colleagues[29] found patients with asymptomatic rotator cuff tears had significantly greater subscapularis activity during internal rotation activities and less upper trapezius activation during carrying activities than symptomatic patients. Also, symptomatic patients had significantly greater supraspinatus, infraspinatus, and upper trapezius muscle activation with shoulder elevation tasks than asymptomatic patients. This information suggests that patients with symptomatic tears continue to fire the torn muscles and attempt to overcompensate with scapular stabilizers compared with asymptomatic patients who use the remainder of the intact cuff.

Symptomatic Full-Thickness Tears

Information regarding the natural history of nonoperatively treated symptomatic rotator cuff tears has been lacking until recently. In general, most information regarding the natural history of symptomatic tears has focused on the clinical outcomes of nonoperatively treated rotator cuff tears.[30–32] Golberg and colleagues[30] evaluated 46 patients treated nonoperatively for symptomatic full-thickness rotator cuff tears with the simple shoulder test at 6-month intervals until an average of 2.5 years after the initial evaluation; 59% of patients experienced functional improvement that remained stable over the follow-up period. Bokor and colleagues[31] evaluated 53 patients at an average of 7.6 years after initial evaluation for a symptomatic full-thickness rotator cuff tear; 74% of patients reported slight or no shoulder discomfort at follow-up although only 56% had a satisfactory UCLA shoulder rating scale. Finally, Hawkins and Dunlop[32] reported on 33 patients at an average of 3.8 years after initial evaluation and found 58% of patients were satisfied. Satisfaction was correlated with improved pain relief and the ability to use the arm at shoulder level. In general, nonoperative treatment of symptomatic full-thickness tears is reasonable, leading to approximately 60% successful results. Although nonoperative treatment can be effective, information regarding who fails conservative treatment and who likely benefits from surgical repair is required to maximize outcomes.

Recently, several articles have been published specifically addressing the clinical and anatomic natural history of nonoperatively treated symptomatic rotator cuff tears. Maman and colleagues[33] evaluated 33 patients with full-thickness symptomatic rotator cuff tears and determined 52% progressed in tear size at an average of 24 months' follow-up. Tear progression was more likely after 18 months (50%) compared with before (19%). Age older than 60 and initial rotator cuff fatty infiltration correlated with tear progression. Safran and colleagues[34] evaluated 51 patients 60 years of age or younger who were treated nonoperatively for a symptomatic full-thickness rotator cuff tear. At an average of 29 months' follow-up, the investigators found an almost identical 49% of tears increased in size (>5 mm). Pain at follow-up was the only factor correlated with tear progression (56% with pain vs 25% without pain; $P = .002$). Conclusions from these articles are that there is a significant risk for tear progression in nonoperatively treated symptomatic full-thickness tears with approximately 50% progressing at an average of 2 years. Due to a high risk for tear progression, early surgical treatment can be considered in young patients with significant (>1–1.5 cm) reparable full-thickness tears without chronic muscle changes because there is a high risk for tear enlargement over time. If tears are to be monitored, then imaging should be performed at 1.5 years or if the shoulder becomes increasingly painful because these factors are correlated with tear progression.

Fucentese and colleagues[35] recently reported on the natural history of symptomatic isolated full-thickness tears. These investigators evaluated 24 patients (average 54 years old) with isolated full-thickness supraspinatus tears at 3.5 years' average follow-up after nonoperative treatment. The average initial tear size was 1.6 cm. Overall, there was no increase in the average tear size at follow-up and only 25% had tear progression in contrast to the 50% reported by Maman and colleagues[33] and Safran and colleagues.[34] They reported no increase in fatty degeneration of the supraspinatus beyond stage 2. Finally, the tear progression that occurred did not affect the reparability of these tears. Consequently, these data suggest that in small (<1–1.5 cm) full-thickness tears, initial observation is reasonable even in young patients, due to a low risk for tear progression (25%) unlike in larger tears, as shown by Maman et al and Safran et al, which have a higher risk (approximately 50%) for tear enlargement.[33–35]

Partial-Thickness Tears

The natural history of nonoperatively treated asymptomatic and symptomatic partial-thickness rotator cuff tears has also been evaluated. Mall and colleagues[25] evaluated 30 asymptomatic partial-thickness rotator cuff tears. At an average of 2-years' follow-up, 20 of the asymptomatic tears that remained asymptomatic were compared with 10 of the tears that became symptomatic. Ultrasound was performed at follow-up to evaluate for tear progression. Looking at the tears remaining asymptomatic, none of these tears progressed to a full-thickness tear. In the 10 tears becoming symptomatic,

40% progressed to a full-thickness tear. Pain was highly correlated with tear progression in asymptomatic partial-thickness tears and, therefore, can be used as a warning sign of enlargement and that further evaluation is warranted, such as a follow-up imaging study.

Maman and colleagues[33] evaluated 30 patients with symptomatic partial-thickness rotator cuff tears at an average of 24 months with an MRI. These investigators found only 10% of symptomatic partial-thickness tears progressed in size (>5 mm), which is significantly less than the 50% progression reported in the same study for symptomatic full-thickness tears. Tear location (bursal-sided or articular-sided) had no affect on tear progression. These data suggest that tear progression of symptomatic partial-thickness tears is at a significantly reduced rate compared with symptomatic full-thickness tears; therefore, initial nonoperative treatment is reasonable due to a decreased risk for tear progression.

ROTATOR CUFF TENDON HEALING
Spontaneous Tendon Healing

The rotator cuff has a limited ability for intrinsic healing without repair. Several investigators have investigated spontaneous rotator cuff healing in animal models.[36–38] No evidence of rotator cuff healing was found at 3 weeks in a 12-mm tear in a rabbit suprapsinatus tear model.[36] Similarly, an active but inadequate repair response was found in a rat supraspinatus tear model where 78% of tendons had persistent defects at 12 weeks after a 2-mm^2 defect was created.[37] The material and structural properties of the reparative tissue was significantly inferior to that of normal tendon.[37] In another rat supraspinatus tear model, only scar tissue was found around tendon stumps after 12 weeks from the time of tendon detachment from the humerus.[38] This evidence suggests a limited potential for spontaneous rotator cuff healing.

Clinical series evaluating patients with partial-thickness and full-thickness rotator cuff tears treated surgically have found limited healing if repair was not performed. In one series, none of the patients treated with arthroscopic débridement and acromioplasty for partial-thickness rotator cuff tears who subsequently underwent second-look arthroscopy had evidence of healing.[39] In another study, there was no evidence of tendon healing as determined by ultrasound at an average of 101 months postoperatively in 26 patients treated with arthroscopic acromioplasty for partial-thickness rotator cuff tears.[40] At the time of follow-up evaluation, 35% of tears progressed from partial thickness to full thickness.[40] Another series showed no patients who underwent revision surgery at an average of 13.7 months after open subacromial decompression for small and medium-sized tears had evidence of healing and 40% had progression of tear size.[41] These studies demonstrate that arthroscopic or open debridement of tears and acromioplasty will not result in spontaneous tendon healing.

Tendon Healing After Repair—Factors Affecting Healing

Even in the setting of rotator cuff repair, complete healing or normal restoration of the tendon insertion is difficult. Investigators have analyzed the ability of the rotator cuff to heal in several animal models. In a rat supraspinatus tendon repair model, repair sites revealed a poor healing response with only partial recreation of the original tendon insertion site by 8 weeks.[42] Biomechanical properties of repaired supraspinatus rat tendons were inferior at 8 weeks after repair compared with uninjured tendon sites.[43,44] Delay in rotator cuff repair has been shown to lead to irreversible rotator cuff muscle changes, including atrophy, fatty infiltration, and impairment of the biomechanical properties of the repair site.[45,46] Therefore, healing after a repair does not recreate a normal tendon insertion and a delay in repair can lead to irreversible changes along with impairment of healing.

The limited ability for normal restoration of a tendon even after repair that was demonstrated in animal studies is reflected in several clinical patient series after rotator cuff repair. Durable long-term clinical results have been proved after rotator cuff repair.[47,48] Despite these excellent clinical results, several reports have suggested that a significant percentage of repairs fail to heal. Single-tendon and 2-tendon retear rates have been reported as 29% and up to 94%, respectively, despite excellent clinical outcomes.[49,50] Failure of tendon healing does not preclude an excellent result, although improved results have been correlated with intact repairs.[51]

Several patient-related biologic factors are important in determining the healing potential of a rotator cuff repair. Patient age, tear size, and tear chronicity are probably the most important biologic factors affecting healing.[49,52,53] Increasing patient age has been correlated with worse healing after open, single-row arthroscopic, and double-row arthroscopic repair.[49,51,54] Boileau and colleagues[49] reported 43% healing in patients over 65 as opposed to 86% healing under age 65 in single tendon tears fixed arthroscopically. Similarly, Tashjian and colleagues[54] and Cho and colleagues[55] determined the average age of unhealed repairs after double-row repair was in the early 60s compared with those that healed was in the mid-50s. There seems to be a tipping point in the early to mid-60s for healing. Several investigators have shown tear size correlates with tendon healing with larger tears having worse healing rates after single-row and double-row rotator cuff repairs.[53,55] Finally, poorer rotator cuff muscle quality has been shown to correlate with worse rotator cuff healing.[56,57] Thomazeau and colleagues[56] reported that worse preoperative atrophy correlated with worse postoperative repair integrity in 30 chronic supraspinatus tears fixed using an open technique. Liem and colleagues[57] recently reported on 53 isolated supraspinatus rotator cuff tears fixed arthroscopically and reported healing correlated with both supraspinatus atrophy and fatty infiltration. They determined that worse preoperative muscle atrophy, similar to Thomazeau and colleagues,[56] correlated with worse healing.[57] Grade 2 or above fatty infiltration was also correlated with worse healing rates.[57]

When biologic factors are favorable (young patients and good muscle quality), then early surgical repair can be considered because healing is more predictable. Older patients or patients with chronic large or massive tears with poor muscle should be considered for early nonoperative treatment because healing is less likely after repair.

INDICATIONS AND TIMING FOR SURGICAL REPAIR

Treatment of rotator cuff tears should be based on the risks and benefits associated with both operative and nonoperative management. The long-term clinical results of both arthroscopic and open rotator cuff repairs are good, with more than 90% good or excellent results at 10 years.[47,58] Similarly, results of nonoperative treatment of rotator cuff tears have shown reasonable success with between 50% and 60% satisfactory results.[30–32] Although most surgeons consider reparability and healing of the tear important for optimal outcome, risk is associated with surgical treatment and repair. Nonoperative treatment is also associated with risks that may be less obvious, but failure to recognize these may lead to potentially avoidable inferior results. Both operative and nonoperative risks are important in considering surgical indications.

The natural history of rotator cuff disease has demonstrated that there are several potential significant risks associated with nonoperative treatment. These risks include a relative lack of spontaneous healing, tear progression, muscle fatty degeneration, tendon retraction, increased difficulty with tendon mobilization, and potential for arthritis. Tear progression has been found in a significant number of patients treated nonoperatively of both symptomatic and asymptomatic tears.[4,33,34] Because increased tear size and poorer muscle quality are associated with poorer healing after surgical repair, repair before progression may improve outcomes.[53,55]

In addition to tear progression, fatty infiltration of the rotator cuff muscles may occur with conservative treatment of tears. Clinical and experimental evidence suggests that infiltration is limited but not reversed by tendon repair.[46,52] Also, increased infiltration at the time of operation predicts poor postoperative results and increased retear rates.[52] Therefore, repair of tears after the development of significant atrophy and fatty infiltration may decrease the overall benefit of surgical repair, altering the overall risk-benefit anaylsis of operative versus nonoperative treatment.

An organized approach for developing operative indications for rotator cuff tears is based on the risks of chronic cuff changes previously described (**Box 1**).[59] Patients are divided into 3 groups taking into consideration the natural history of partial-thickness and full-thickness tears, the potential for repair healing, the reparability of the tear, and various postoperative outcome factors. Categorization of patients is as follows: group I, minimal risk for chronic rotator cuff changes in the near future; group II, significant risk for irreversible changes to the rotator cuff with prolonged therapy and nonoperative care and a high capacity for rotator cuff healing; and group III, chronic rotator cuff and articular cartilage changes are already present or limited capacity for rotator cuff healing after repair. Based on these groups, the indications for early repair of a tear can be delineated.

Group I—Rotator Cuff Tendonitis, Partial-Thickness Tears (Except Larger Bursal-Sided Tears), and Small (<1–1.5 cm) Full-Thickness Tears

Prolonged physical therapy and nonoperative treatment should be considered in patients with rotator cuff tendonitis, partial-thickness tears (except maybe larger bursal-sided tears), and potentially small full-thickness tears. There is limited risk for the development of irreversible, chronic changes, such as fatty infiltration, tendon retraction, or glenohumeral arthritis with this treatment regimen.

Although there are no data on the incidence of tear progression in patients with rotator cuff tendonitis, the likelihood is probably low. Nonoperative treatment of

---

Box 1
Treatment algorithm for rotator cuff disease

- Group I—initial nonoperative treatment
  - Tendonitis
  - Partial-thickness tears (except maybe larger bursal-sided tears)
  - Maybe small (<1 cm) full-thickness tears
- Group II—consider early surgical repair
  - All acute tears full-thickness (except maybe small [<1 cm] tears)
  - All chronic full-thickness tears in a young (<65) age group (except maybe small [<1 cm] tears)
- Group III—initial nonoperative treatment
  - All chronic full-thickness tears in an older (>65 or 70) age group
  - Irreparable tears (based on tear size, retraction, muscle quality, and migration)

rotator cuff tendonitis or impingement syndrome (intact rotator cuff) has been shown to have a high success rate, with between 61% and 67% of patients having a satisfactory result at greater than 2 years.[60,61] Similarly, 2 prospective, randomized controlled studies have found significant improvements in patients with subacromial impingement after both subacromial decompression and supervised physiotherapy. No significant differences, however, were found between the 2 treatments.[60,62] Based on the results of these studies, prolonged nonoperative treatment is recommended for patients with rotator cuff tendonitis.

Initial conservative treatment is also recommended for most partial-thickness rotator cuff tears. Although healing has not been shown to occur with partial tears without repair, significant improvements in functional outcomes have been shown with conservative treatment.[40,63] Similarly, there has been shown to be a slow, small risk for tear progression.[25,33] The only exception may be larger bursal-sided partial-thickness tears, which have been shown to not respond as well to physical therapy and subacromial decompression as articular-sided tears.[64,65] Thus, although the authors generally recommend prolonged conservative treatment for partial-thickness tears, earlier repair may be indicated in large bursal-sided partial tears secondary to higher failure rates of nonoperative treatment.

Finally, Fucentese and colleagues[35] have recently shown a low rate of tear progression for small (<1 cm–1.5 cm) full-thickness tears. Consequently, initial nonoperative treatment is reasonable to consider in both acute and chronic small (<1 cm–1.5 cm) full-thickness tears independent of age due to the small risk for progression. If observation is performed, then an MRI should be performed at 12 to 18 months from evaluation or if symptoms progress to monitor for tear progression.[33,34]

Prolonged nonoperative treatment is reasonable in this category (group I) due to the limited risk for irreversible, chronic rotator cuff changes.

Group II—Any Acute Full-Thickness Tear or Any Chronic Full-Thickness Tear in a Young (<65-Year-Old) Age Group (Except Possibly Small [<1–1.5 cm] Full-Thickness Tears)

Group II is comprised of patients younger than 65 years old with chronic full-thickness tears and acute tears in any age group excluding patients with small (<1–1.5 cm) full-thickness tears. Early surgical intervention is warranted in this category (group II) due to significant risks for irreversible changes with nonoperative treatment and a high likelihood of healing if repair is performed.

Several investigators have described absolute indications for operative intervention for acute full-thickness rotator cuff tears. Mantone and colleagues[66] have indicated that patients younger than 50 years old with acute rotator cuff tears should undergo early operative fixation. Wirth and colleagues[67] has recommended repair instead of initial conservative treatment in active patients with acute tears after trauma. Bassett and Cofield[68] have recommended repair within 3 weeks of acute tears for maximal restoration of shoulder function, specifically improved shoulder abduction. More recently, Bjornsson and colleagues[69] have determined that no significant differences in tendon healing, pain, shoulder elevation, or functional outcomes occur if an acute tear was fixed within 3 months of injury compared with within 3 weeks. Petersen and Murphy[70] reported that patients with acute tears fixed after 4 months had worse American Shoulder and Elbow Surgeons scores, active forward elevation, and satisfaction than if fixed before 4 months. Based on this information, substantial (>1–1.5 cm) acute full-thickness tears are recommended to be fixed early within the first 3 to 4 months with no apparent effect on healing or outcomes if fixed within this time period.

All young (<65 years old) patients with substantial (>1–1.5 cm) full-thickness tears without significant muscle deterioration can also be considered for early surgical repair. Based on natural history data of Maman and colleagues[33] and Safran and colleagues,[34] there is a significant risk tear progression in this group. Tear progression includes tear extension, fatty changes of the rotator cuff muscles, and tendon retraction. Repair should be considered not only because of a high rate of tear progression but also because healing data support improved healing rates in this same group, as described previously.[49,51,54] Small full-thickness tears (<1–1.5 cm) have a limited risk for tear progression; therefore, these smaller tears can be considered for initial nonoperative treatment compared with larger tears.[35]

Group III—Chronic Full-thickness Tears in Older Patients (>65 or 70) or Irreparable Tears with Significant Irreversible Changes Present

Group III comprises older patients over age 65 or 70 with chronic full-thickness rotator cuff tears or individuals of any age with large or massive rotator cuff tears with chronic, irreversible rotator cuff changes already present. Initial nonoperative treatment for this group is recommended.

In the setting of large or massive tears with chronic irreversible changes to the rotator cuff muscle, the risks of nonoperative treatment are small because most of these injuries are irreparable. Several factors have been identified on imaging studies that correlate with irreparability. Sugihara and colleagues[71] determined that tears greater than 4 cm in width and length and severe fatty infiltration of the supraspinatus (grade 3 or 4) and infraspinatus on preoperative MRIs correlated with irreparability. Static superior humeral head migration on plain radiographs is also a marker for irreparability as a reduced acromiohumeral index has been correlated with massive tears, fatty degeneration of the supraspinatus and infraspinatus and very chronic tears (older than 5 years).[72] Therefore, large and massive cuff tears with severe grade 3 or 4 fatty infiltration of the rotator cuff with a narrowed acromiohumeral index on plain films can be considered irreparable and treated with initial prolonged nonoperative treatment.

In the case of older patients, healing of a rotator cuff tear is unlikely even after repair. Only 43% of patients over age 65 treated with arthroscopic rotator cuff repair of a full-thickness supraspinatus tear had evidence of healing at 18 months postoperatively compared with 86% of patients under age 65.[49] Despite limited healing, arthroscopic repairs in elderly patients is feasible with one group demonstrating that 80% of patients over age 60 had satisfactory clinical results independent of tear size or the ability to complete the repair by only performing margin convergence.[73] Because healing is unlikely, the goal of surgery in elderly patients may be to convert a symptomatic tear to an asymptomatic tear. Consequently, the risk of tear progression may be less important because a complete repair is not required or feasible due to limited healing potential.

A prolonged trial of therapy is reasonable in these cases (group III) before consideration of surgical treatment.

SUMMARY

The etiology of rotator cuff disease is likely multifactorial, including age-related degeneration and microtrauma and macrotrauma. The incidence of rotator cuff tears increases with aging with more than half of individuals in their 80s having a rotator cuff tear. Smoking, hypercholesterolemia, and genetics have all been shown to influence the development of rotator cuff tearing. Substantial full-thickness rotator cuff tears, in general, progress and enlarge with time. Pain, or worsening pain, usually signals tear progression in both asymptomatic and symptomatic tears and should warrant further investigation if the tear is treated conservatively. Larger (>1–1.5 cm) symptomatic full-thickness cuff tears have a high rate of tear progression and, therefore, should be considered for earlier surgical repair in younger patients if the tear is reparable and there is limited muscle degeneration to avoid irreversible changes to the cuff, including tear enlargement and degenerative muscle changes. Smaller symptomatic full-thickness tears have been shown to have a slower rate of progression, similar to partial-thickness tears, and can be considered for initial nonoperative treatment due to the limited risk for rapid tear progression. In both small full-thickness tears and partial-thickness tears, increasing pain should alert physicians to obtain further imaging as it can signal tear progression.

Natural history data, along with information on factors affecting healing after rotator cuff repair, can help guide surgeons in making appropriate decisions regarding the treatment of rotator cuff tears. The management of rotator cuff tears should be considered in the context of the risks and benefits of operative versus nonoperative treatment. Tear size and acuity, the presence of irreparable changes to the rotator cuff or glenohumeral joint, and patient age should all be considered in making this decision. Initial nonoperative care can be safely undertaken in older patients (>70 years old) with chronic tears; in patients with irreparable rotator cuff tears with irreversible changes, including significant atrophy and fatty infiltration, humeral head migration, and arthritis; in patients of any age with small (<1 cm) full-thickness tears; or in patients without a full-thickness tear. Early surgical treatment can be considered in significant (>1 cm–1.5 cm) acute tears or young patients with full-thickness tears who have a significant risk for the development of irreparable rotator cuff changes.

REFERENCES

1. Chakravarty K, Webley M. Shoulder joint movement and its relationship to disability in the elderly. J Rheumatol 1993;20:1359–61.
2. Dunn WR, Schackman BR, Walsh C, et al. Variation in orthopaedic surgeons' perceptions about the indications for rotator cuff surgery. J Bone Joint Surg Am 2005;87:1978–84.
3. Duckworth DG, Smith KL, Campbell B, et al. Self-assessment questionnaires document substantial variability in the clinical expression of rotator cuff tears. J Shoulder Elbow Surg 1999;8(4):330–3.
4. Yamaguchi K, Tetro AM, Blam O, et al. Natural history of asymptomatic rotator cuff tears: a longitudinal analysis of asymptomatic tears detected sonographically. J Shoulder Elbow Surg 2001;10:199–203.
5. Matsen FA, Titelman RM, Lippitt SB, et al. Rotator cuff. In: Rockwood CA, Matsen FA, Wirth MA, et al, editors. The Shoulder. Philadelphia: WB Saunders; 2004. p. 795–878.
6. Neer CS. Impingement lesions. Clin Orthop 1983;173:70–7.
7. Lehman C, Cuomo F, Kummer FJ, et al. The incidence of full thickness rotator cuff tears in a large cadaveric population. Bull Hosp Jt Dis 1995;54(1):30–1.
8. Yamanaka K, Fukada H. Pathologic studies of the supraspinatus tendon with reference to incomplete partial thickness tear. In: Takagishi N, editor. The Shoulder. Tokyo: Professional Postgraduate Services; 1987. p. 220–4.
9. Sher JS, Uribe JW, Posada A, et al. Abnormal findings on magnetic resonance images of asymptomatic shoulders. J Bone Joint Surg Am 1995;77:10–5.
10. Tempelhof S, Rupp S, Seil R. Age-related prevalence of rotator cuff tears in asymptomatic shoulders. J Shoulder Elbow Surg 1999;8:296–9.

11. Yamaguchi K, Ditsios K, Middleton WD, et al. The demographic and morphological features of rotator cuff disease. A comparison of asymptomatic and symptomatic shoulders. J Bone Joint Surg Am 2006;88(8):1699–704.
12. Yamamoto A, Takagishi K, Osawa T, et al. Prevalence and risk factors of a rotator cuff tear in the general population. J Shoulder Elbow Surg 2010;19(1):116–20.
13. Katzer A, Wening JV, Becker-Mannich HU, et al. Rotator cuff rupture. Vascular supply and collagen fiber processes as pathogenetic factors. Unfallchirurgie 1997;23:52–9.
14. Mosley LH, Finseth F. Cigarette smoking: impairment of digital blood flow and wound healing in the hand. Hand 1977;9:97–101.
15. Blevins F, Djurasovic M, Flatow E, et al. Biology of the rotator cuff. Orthop Clin North Am 1997;28:1–15.
16. Baumgarten KM, Gerlack D, Galatz LM, et al. Cigarette smoking increases the risk for rotator cuff tears. Clin Orthop Relat Res 2010;468:1534–41.
17. Carbone S, Gumina S, Arceri V, et al. The impact of preoperative smoking habit on rotator cuff tear: cigarette smoking influences rotator cuff tear sizes. J Shoulder Elbow Surg 2012;21:56–60.
18. Galatz LM, Silva MJ, Rothermich SY, et al. Nicotine delays tendon-to-bone healing in a rat shoulder model. J Bone Joint Surg Am 2006;88(9):2027–34.
19. Mallon WJ, Misamore G, Snead DS, et al. The impact of preoperative smoking habits on the results of rotator cuff repair. J Shoulder Elbow Surg 2004;13(2):129–32.
20. Beason DP, Abboud JA, Kuntz AF, et al. Cumulative effects of hypercholesterolemia on tendon biomechanics in a mouse model. J Orthop Res 2011;29:380–3.
21. Abboud JA, Kim JS. The effect of hypercholesterolemia on rotator cuff disease. Clin Orthop Relat Res 2010;468:1493–7.
22. Harvie P, Ostlere SJ, Teh J, et al. Genetic influences in the aetiology of tears of the rotator cuff. Sibling risk of a full-thickness tear. J Bone Joint Surg Br 2004;86(5):696–700.
23. Gwilym SE, Watkins B, Cooper CD, et al. Genetic influences in the progression of tears of the rotator cuff. J Bone Joint Surg Br 2009;91(7):915–7.
24. Tashjian RZ, Farnham JM, Albright FS, et al. Evidence for an inherited predisposition contributing to the risk for rotator cuff disease. J Bone Joint Surg Am 2009;91(5):1136–42.
25. Mall NA, Kim HM, Keener JD, et al. Symptomatic progression of asymptomatic rotator cuff tears: a prospective study of clinical and sonographic variables. J Bone Joint Surg Am 2010;92(16):2623–33.
26. Burkhart SS. Flouroscopic comparison of kinematic patterns in massive rotator cuff tears. A suspension bridge model. Clin Orthop Relat Res 1992;284:144–52.
27. Yamaguchi K, Sher JS, Andersen WK, et al. Glenohumeral motion in patients with rotator cuff tears: a comparison of asymptomatic and symptomatic shoulders. J Shoulder Elbow Surg 2000;9:6–11.
28. Keener JD, Wei AS, Kim M, et al. Proximal humeral migration in shoulders with symptomatic and asymptomatic rotator cuff tears. J Bone Joint Surg Am 2009;91(6):1405–13.
29. Kelly BT, Williams RJ, Cordasco FA, et al. Differential patterns of muscle activation in patients with symptomatic and asymptomatic rotator cuff tears. J Shoulder Elbow Surg 2005;14:165–71.
30. Goldberg BA, Nowinski RJ, Matsen FA 3rd. Outcome of nonoperative management of full-thickness rotator cuff tears. Clin Orthop Relat Res 2001;382:99–107.

31. Bokor DJ, Hawkins RJ, Huckell GH, et al. Results of nonoperative management of full-thickness tears of the rotator cuff. Clin Orthop Relat Res 1993;294:103–10.
32. Hawkins RH, Dunlop R. Nonoperative treatment of rotator cuff tears. Clin Orthop Relat Res 1995;321:178–88.
33. Maman E, Harris C, White L, et al. Outcome of nonoperative treatment of symptomatic rotator cuff tears monitored by magnetic resonance imaging. J Bone Joint Surg Am 2009;91(8):1898–906.
34. Safran O, Schroeder J, Bloom R, et al. Natural history of nonoperatively treated symptomatic rotator cuff tears in patients 60 years old or younger. Am J Sports Med 2011;39(4):710–4.
35. Fucentese SF, von Roll AL, Pfirrmann CW, et al. Evolution of nonoperatively treated symptomatic isolated full-thickness supraspinatus tears. J Bone Joint Surg 2012;94:801–8.
36. Hirose K, Kondo S, Choi H, et al. Spontaneous healing process of a supraspinatus tendon tear in rabbits. Arch Orthop Trauma Surg 2004;124:374–7.
37. Carpenter JE, Thomopoulos S, Flanagan CL, et al. Rotator cuff defect healing: a biomechanical and histologic analysis in an animal model. J Shoulder Elbow Surg 1998;7:599–605.
38. Gimbel JA, Mehta S, Van Kleunen JP, et al. The tension required at repair to reappose the supraspinatus tendon to bone rapidly increases after injury. Clin Orthop 2004;426:258–65.
39. Weber SC. Arthroscopic debridement and acromioplasty versus mini-open repair in the treatment of significant partial-thickness rotator cuff tears. Arthroscopy 1999;15:126–31.
40. Kartus J, Kartus C, Rostgard-Christensen L, et al. Long-terms clinical and ultrasound evaluation after arthroscopic acromioplasty in patients with partial rotator cuff tears. Arthroscopy 2006;22:44–9.
41. Massoud SN, Levy O, Copeland SA. Subacromial decompression. Treatment for small- and medium-sized tears of the rotator cuff. J Bone Joint Surg Br 2002;84:955–60.
42. Thomopoulos S, Hattersley G, Rosen V, et al. The localized expression of extracellular matrix components in healing tendon insertion sites: an in situ hybridization study. J Orthop Res 2002;20:454–63.
43. Galatz LM, Sandell LJ, Rothermich SY, et al. Characteristics of the rat supraspinatus tendon during tendon-to-bone healing after acute injury. J Orthop Res 2006;24:541–50.
44. Thomopoulos S, Williams GR, Gimbel JA, et al. Variation of biomechanical, structural, and compositional properties along the tendon to bone insertion site. J Orthop Res 2003;21:413–9.
45. Galatz LM, Rothermich SY, Zaegel M, et al. Delayed repair of tendon to bone injuries leads to decreased biomechanical properties and bone loss. J Orthop Res 2005;23:1441–7.
46. Gerber C, Meyer DC, Schneeberger AG, et al. Effect of tendon release and delayed repair on the structure of the muscles of the rotator cuff: an experimental study in sheep. J Bone Joint Surg Am 2004;86:1973–82.
47. Galatz LM, Griggs S, Cameron BD, et al. Prospective longitudinal analysis of postoperative shoulder function: a ten-year follow-up study of full-thickness rotator cuff tears. J Bone Joint Surg Am 2001;83:1052–6.
48. Zandi H, Coghlan JA, Bell SN. Mini-incision rotator cuff repair: a longitudinal assessment with no deterioration of result up to nine years. J Shoulder Elbow Surg 2006;15:135–9.

49. Boileau P, Brassart N, Watkinson DJ, et al. Arthroscopic repair of full-thickness tears of the supraspinatus: does the tendon really heal? J Bone Joint Surg Am 2005;87:1229–40.

50. Galatz LM, Ball CM, Teefey SA, et al. The outcome and repair integrity of completely arthroscopically repaired large and massive rotator cuff tears. J Bone Joint Surg Am 2004;86:219–24.

51. Harryman DT, Mack LA, Wang KY, et al. Repairs of the rotator cuff. Correlation of functional results with integrity of the cuff. J Bone Joint Surg Am 1991;73:982–9.

52. Goutallier D, Postel JM, Gleyze P, et al. Influence of cuff muscle fatty degeneration on anatomic and functional outcomes after simple suture of full-thickness tears. J Shoulder Elbow Surg 2003;12:550–4.

53. Gulotta LV, Nho SJ, Dodson CC, et al. Prospective evaluation of arthroscopic rotator cuff repairs at 5 years: part II – prognostic factors for clinical and radiographic outcomes. J Shoulder Elbow Surg 2011;20:941–6.

54. Tashjian RZ, Hollins AM, Kim HM, et al. Factors affecting healing rates after arthroscopic double-row rotator cuff repair. Am J Sports Med 2010;38:2435–42.

55. Cho NS, Lee BG, Rhee YG. Arthroscopic rotator cuff repair using a suture bridge technique. Is the repair integrity actually maintained? Am J Sports Med 2011;39:2108–16.

56. Thomazeau H, Boukobza E, Morcet N, et al. Prediction of rotator cuff repair results by magnetic resonance imaging. Clin Orthop Relat Res 1997;344:275–83.

57. Liem D, Lichtenberg S, Magosch P, et al. Magnetic resonance imaging of arthroscopic supraspinatus tendon repair. J Bone Joint Surg Am 2007;89:1770–6.

58. Wolf EM, Pennington WT, Agrawal V. Arthroscopic rotator cuff repair: 4- to 10-year results. Arthroscopy 2004;20:5–12.

59. Lashgari CJ, Yamaguchi K. Natural history and nonsurgical treatment of rotator cuff disorders. In: Norris TR, editor. Orthopaedic knowledge update: shoulder and elbow 2. Rosemont (IL): American Academy of Orthopaedic Surgeons; 2002. p. 155–62.

60. Brox JI, Gjengendal E, Uppheim G, et al. Arthroscopic surgery versus supervised exercises in patients with rotator cuff disease (stage II impingement syndrome): a prospective, randomized, controlled study in 125 patients with a 2 ½ - year follow-up. J Shoulder Elbow Surg 1999;8:102–11.

61. Morrison DS, Frogameni AD, Woodworth P. Non-operative treatment of subacromial impingement syndrome. J Bone Joint Surg Am 1997;79:732–7.

62. Haahr JP, Ostergaard S, Dalsgaard J, et al. Exercises versus arthroscopic decompression in patients with subacromial impingement: a randomized, controlled study in 90 cases with a one year follow up. Ann Rheum Dis 2005;64:760–4.

63. Yamanaka K, Matsumoto T. The joint side tear of the rotator cuff. A followup study by arthrography. Clin Orthop 1994;304:68–73.

64. Fukada H, Hamada K, Nakajima T, et al. Partial-thickness tears of the rotator cuff; a clinicopathological review based on 66 surgically verified cases. Int Orthop 1996;20:257–65.

65. Cordasco FA, Backer M, Craig EV, et al. The partial-thickness rotator cuff tear: is acromioplasty without repair sufficient? Am J Sports Med 2002;30:257–60.

66. Mantone JK, Burkhead WZ, Noonan J. Nonoperative treatment of rotator cuff tears. Orthop Clin North Am 2000;31:295–311.

67. Wirth MA, Basamania C, Rockwood CA. Nonoperative management of full-thickness tears of the rotator cuff. Orthop Clin North Am 1997;28:59–67.

68. Bassett RW, Cofield RH. Acute tears of the rotator cuff. The timing of surgical repair. Clin Orthop 1983;175:18–24.
69. Bjornsson HC, Norlin R, Johansson K, et al. The influence of age, delay of repair, and tendon involvement in acute rotator cuff tears: structural and clinical outcomes after repair of 42 shoulders. Acta Orthop 2011;82(2):187–92.
70. Petersen SA, Murphy TP. The timing of rotator cuff repair for the restoration of function. J Shoulder Elbow Surg 2011;20(1):62–8.
71. Sugihara T, Nakagawa T, Tsuchiya M, et al. Prediction of primary reparability of massive tears of the rotator cuff on preoperative magnetic resonance imaging. J Shoulder Elbow Surg 2003;12(3):222–5.
72. Nove-Josserand L, Edwards TB, O'Connor DP, et al. The acromiohumeral and coracohumeral intervals are abnormal in rotator cuff tears with muscle fatty degeneration. Clin Orthop Relat Res 2005;433:90–6.
73. Rebuzzi E, Coletti N, Schiavetti S, et al. Arthroscopic rotator cuff repair in patients older than 60 years. Arthroscopy 2005;21:48–54.

Imaging Evaluation of the Rotator Cuff

Mark W. Anderson, MD*, Christopher Brennan, MD,
Amit Mittal, MD

KEYWORDS

- Rotator cuff • Imaging • Radiography • Computed tomography
- Magnetic resonance imaging

KEY POINTS

- Imaging plays an important role in the workup of a patient with suspected rotator cuff abnormality.
- Radiographs should be the first imaging study obtained, and may reveal anatomic features that predispose to rotator cuff abnormality or secondary signs of a rotator cuff tear.
- Magnetic resonance (MR) imaging provides the best overall evaluation of the cuff, and MR arthrography is especially helpful for detecting subtle cuff abnormality.
- Computed tomographic arthrography provides an excellent alternative for patients who are unable to undergo MR imaging or for assessing the postoperative cuff when metallic hardware has been used in a prior repair.

ANATOMIC CONSIDERATIONS
Gross Anatomy

The rotator cuff is a complex, multilayered structure formed by the confluence of the supraspinatus, infraspinatus, teres minor, and subscapularis tendons (**Fig. 1**). Superficial fibers are uniform and distinct while deep fibers are interwoven to provide increased strength and glenohumeral joint stability.[1] The supraspinatus muscle initiates the first 15° to 30° of arm abduction while the infraspinatus and teres minor muscles externally rotate the shoulder. The subscapularis muscle adducts and internally rotates the shoulder.

The supraspinatus muscle is made up of 2 components: a fusiform muscle belly arising anteriorly from the supraspinatus fossa, and a unipennate muscle originating posteriorly from the scapular spine.[2] Muscle fibers course laterally, passing beneath the acromioclavicular (AC) joint to form a unified tendon that inserts almost entirely

The University of Virginia Health Sciences Center, Charlottesville, VA 22908-0170, USA
* Corresponding author. Department of Radiology, University of Virginia Health Sciences Center, 1218 Lee Street, Charlottesville, VA 22908-0170, USA.
E-mail address: mwa3a@virginia.edu

Clin Sports Med 31 (2012) 605–631
http://dx.doi.org/10.1016/j.csm.2012.07.010
0278-5919/12/$ – see front matter © 2012 Elsevier Inc. All rights reserved.
sportsmed.theclinics.com

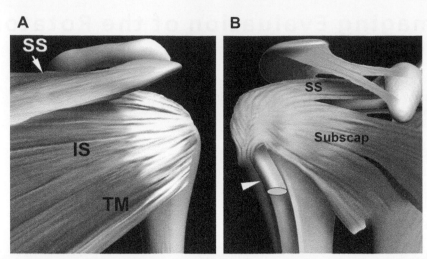

Fig. 1. Rotator cuff muscles along the posterior (*A*) and anterior (*B*) aspects of the joint (*Arrowhead* = long head of the biceps tendon). IS, infraspinatus; SS (*arrow* in *A*), supraspinatus; Subscap, subscapularis; TM, teres minor.

on the superior (horizontal) facet along the anterior portion of the greater tuberosity. Other tendon fibers merge anteriorly with the coracohumeral ligament and posteroinferiorly with the anterior fibers of the infraspinatus tendon.[3] The supraspinatus is supplied by the suprascapular artery and nerve that course just deep to the muscle along suprascapular fossa to the spinoglenoid notch.

The infraspinatus muscle originates from the infraspinatus fossa, and is supplied by distal fibers of the suprascapular nerve as they emerge from the spinoglenoid notch. Multipennate muscle fibers demonstrate a fan-like distribution and converge posterosuperiorly where its tendon inserts on the middle (angled) facet of the greater tuberosity. Deep tendon fibers mesh superiorly with the supraspinatus tendon and inferiorly with the teres minor tendon.

The teres minor muscle originates from the upper two-thirds of the lateral scapula and courses anterior-superiorly. Its tendon blends with the posterior joint capsule and inserts onto the inferior (vertical) facet along the posterior aspect of the greater tuberosity. The muscle forms the superior border of the quadrilateral space, which contains the axillary nerve and circumflex humeral vessels. Additional boundaries of the quadrilateral space include the teres major inferiorly, the long head of the triceps medially, and the humeral shaft laterally.

The subscapularis is a multipennate muscle arising from the subscapular fossa along the anterior surface of the scapula. Most of the fibers of the subscapularis tendon insert on the lesser tuberosity; however, some interdigitate with the coracohumeral/superior glenohumeral ligament and supraspinatus tendon to form an annular structure that ensheaths the long head of the biceps tendon at the level of the proximal bicipital groove (**Fig. 2**). Numerous cadaveric studies suggest that this complex represents what traditionally has been referred to as the transverse humeral ligament.[4,5] Traumatic injury to these components may result in biceps tendon instability.

The "footprint" of each rotator cuff tendon is an important anatomic concept. Each tendon has an articular surface facing the joint, a nonarticular (bursal) surface and a footprint between the two where the tendon attaches to the humerus (**Fig. 3**).[6] The cuff tendons are reinforced near their insertions by fibrocartilage that varies in

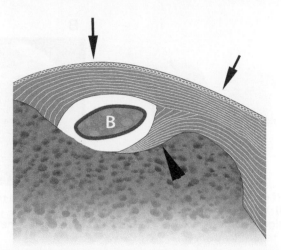

Fig. 2. The "transverse" ligament. Distal insertion of the subscapularis tendon in the axial plane demonstrates tendon fibers coursing both anterior (*arrows*) and posterior (*arrowhead*) to the long head of the biceps tendon (B) within the bicipital groove.

quantity along the width of each tendon.[7] The fibrocartilage provides a 2-layered defense mechanism to protect the tendon with a superficial, nonmineralized portion preventing fiber bending, splitting, and compression, and a deeper calcified fibrocartilage portion that anchors the tendon to bone. Blood vessels do not traverse the fibrocartilage plug, contributing to poor tendon vascularity in this region.

Another important anatomic feature is the rotator cuff cable: a thickened band of collagen fibers that runs perpendicular to the long axis of the supraspinatus and infraspinatus tendons approximately 1 to 2 cm proximal to their insertion sites.[8] It extends from the anterior margin of the supraspinatus tendon posteriorly across the infraspinatus tendon, with both ends affixed to the humeral head. The portion of the cuff lateral to the cable is known as the rotator crescent (**Fig. 4**). Experimental studies using tensile loading suggest symbiotic stabilizing roles of the crescent and cable. The rotator cuff cable has been likened to the cable of a suspension bridge, and likely serves to distribute forces uniformly across the cuff. It may also provide a "rip-stop"

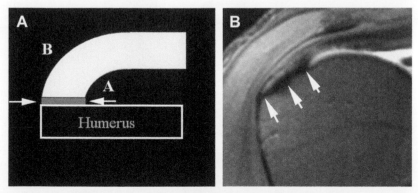

Fig. 3. Rotator cuff footprint. (*A*) Diagram of a rotator cuff tendon demonstrates its articular (A) and bursal (B) surfaces as well as its "footprint," where it inserts on the humerus (between *arrows*). (*B*) Oblique coronal fat-saturated T1-weighted image (MR arthrogram) displays the low-signal "footprint" of the supraspinatus tendon (*arrows*).

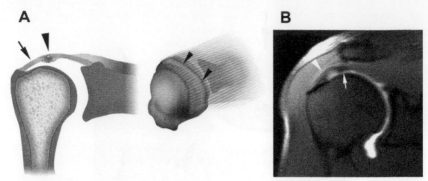

Fig. 4. Rotator cuff cable. (*A*) The rotator cuff "cable" (*arrowheads*) and rotator cuff "crescent" (*arrow*). (*B*) Oblique coronal fat-saturated T1-weighted image (MR arthrogram) displays the low-signal-intensity cable in cross section (*arrow*) along the undersurface of the supraspinatus tendon (*arrowhead*).

mechanism for limiting the extent of rotator cuff tear in some patients. If anterior and posterior cable attachments remain intact despite tearing of the distal (crescent) fibers, glenohumeral function may be preserved secondary to the cable's ability to provide adequate stabilization (force coupling) of the humerus. Based on the prevailing structure, rotator cuffs may be classified as crescent-dominant or cable-dominant.[8,9]

The "outlet" (coracoacromial arch) of the shoulder is an anatomic space formed by the humeral head posteriorly and inferiorly, the acromion and distal clavicle (forming the acromioclavicular joint) superiorly, and the coracoid process and coracoacromial ligament anterior-superiorly (**Fig. 5**). The supraspinatus muscle and tendon course

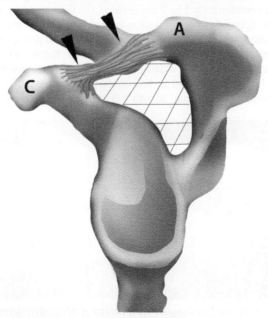

Fig. 5. "Outlet" of the shoulder. Diagram in an oblique sagittal plane demonstrating the outlet of the shoulder (crosshatched area) between the acromion (A), coracoid (C), the intervening coracoacromial ligament (*arrowheads*), and glenoid.

through this space on their way to insert on the greater tuberosity. Anything that decreases this space such as AC joint hypertrophy, abnormal acromial morphology or spurring, or thickening of the coracoacromial ligament may result in symptoms of cuff impingement.

The rotator interval is a triangular space that lies between the anterior border of the supraspinatus tendon, the superior margin of the subscapularis tendon, and the cora-coid process (**Fig. 6**).[10] The floor is formed by the articular surface of the humeral head while the roof is formed by capsule containing the coracohumeral ligament. The cor-acohumeral ligament courses laterally, where it merges with the superior glenohum-eral ligament to form a suspensory sling anteriorly that supports the long head of the biceps tendon as it courses into the bicipital groove.[11] When this anterior biceps "pulley" is torn, the biceps tendon may sublux out of the groove and become entrap-ped between the humeral head and acromion or coracoacromial ligament,[12] explain-ing why anterior supraspinatus tears extending into the rotator interval often result in concomitant biceps tendon abnormality.

Imaging Anatomy

Magnetic resonance imaging and computed tomographic arthrography

Because of their orientation, the supraspinatus and infraspinatus tendons are best demonstrated on coronal and sagittal images that are oriented to the long axis of the supraspinatus muscle (**Fig. 7**). The oblique coronal plane is especially useful for assessing the footprints of the tendons along the greater tuberosity. Oblique sagittal images provide the best demonstration of the structures of the coracoacromial arch and rotator cuff interval as well as the teres minor tendon, all of which are displayed in cross section in this plane (**Fig. 8**). The subscapularis muscle and tendon, as well as the bicipital groove, are best evaluated on axial images (**Fig. 9**).

IMAGING OPTIONS
Radiography

Imaging evaluation of the shoulder begins with conventional radiographs, which are inexpensive, easy to obtain, and allow for evaluation of osseous abnormalities while providing secondary information about soft-tissue abnormality. Numerous radio-graphic views may be obtained depending on the clinical concern, including specific

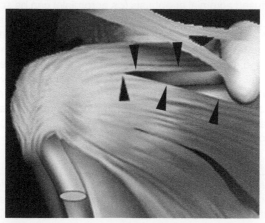

Fig. 6. The rotator cuff interval (*arrowheads*) lies between the supraspinatus and subscapu-laris tendons. Note that the long head of the biceps courses through the interval.

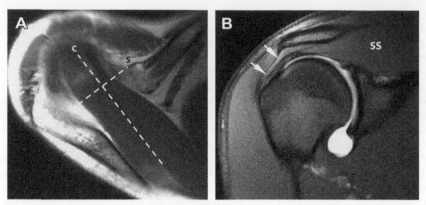

Fig. 7. MR imaging planes. (A) Axial T1-weighted image at the level of the supraspinatus muscle, with dashed lines indicating the scanning planes used for acquiring oblique coronal (C) and oblique sagittal (S) images of the shoulder. (B) Fat-saturated T1-weighted image (MR arthrogram) obtained in the oblique coronal plane shows long-axis demonstration of the supraspinatus muscle (SS) and tendon (arrows).

views that assist in identifying osseous abnormalities that contribute to rotator cuff impingement.[13]

Anteroposterior (AP) views are obtained with the x-ray beam passing through the patient from anterior to posterior, centered at the shoulder. The arm may be held in a neutral, adducted position or with the humerus internally or externally rotated (**Fig. 10**). An AP view is helpful for assessing acromioclavicular joint width, undersurface spurring, lateral tilt of the acromion, and the distance between the humeral head and anterior acromion. A Grashey projection is an AP view with the tube angled to profile the glenohumeral joint (see **Fig. 10**).

An active abduction view is similar to a true AP view except that the arm of the patient is abducted to 90°. This view is also used to assess the humeral-acromial distance (see **Fig. 10**).[14]

An axillary view is centered over the axilla with the arm abducted and the x-ray beam passing cranially through the shoulder (**Fig. 11**). The coracohumeral distance and the presence of an unfused acromial apophysis (os acromiale) can be seen with this view.

The outlet view is obtained with the anterolateral aspect of the affected shoulder placed against the x-ray plate or image receptor, and the beam directed from posterior to anterior along the scapular spine with a 10° caudal tilt. The morphology of the acromion (flat, curved, hooked) is best assessed with this view (see **Fig. 11**).

The acromion may also be evaluated on the Stryker notch view, although this is more typically performed to evaluate for a Hill-Sachs lesion after a dislocation. For this view, the patient is supine and a detector is placed under the affected shoulder. The palm is placed on the forehead and the beam is centered over the coracoid process with 10° of cephalad angulation.

Ultrasonography

Ultrasonography has been reported to be an accurate method for assessing the rotator cuff tendons and for detecting full-thickness and, to a lesser degree, partial-thickness cuff tears.[15–18] Compared with computed tomography (CT) and magnetic resonance (MR) imaging, advantages of ultrasonography include its portability, lower cost, lack of ionizing radiation, and ability to perform real-time, dynamic imaging of the

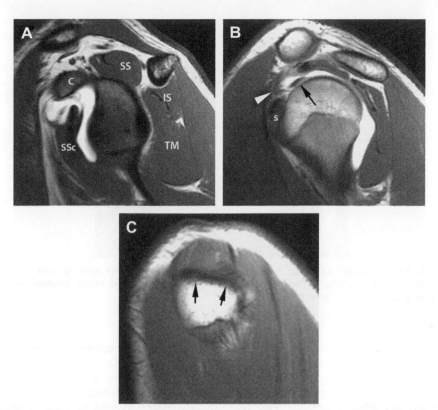

Fig. 8. Oblique sagittal images. (*A*) At the level of the glenoid and coracoid (C), the rotator cuff muscles are seen in cross section. IS, infraspinatus; SSc, subscapularis; SS, supraspinatus; TM, teres minor. (*B*) At a more lateral level, the biceps tendon (*arrow*) is seen as it courses through the rotator cuff interval. The coracohumeral and superior glenohumeral ligaments merge to form the biceps "sling" (*arrowhead*) along the superior margin of the subscapularis (S). (*C*) At a far lateral image, the terminal fibers of the supraspinatus and infraspinatus tendons attach to the greater tuberosity (*arrows*) producing the "hair on the head" pattern of a normal cuff insertion.

shoulder.[18] Variable image quality related to the operator dependence of the technique coupled with limited evaluation of the labrum and bone has prevented the widespread use of this technique in the United States, and it is not be further addressed in this article.

Computed Tomography

CT of the shoulder is typically performed with the patient lying supine within the scanner with the arm adducted and externally rotated. Scanning is typically performed in the axial plane. Submillimeter slice thickness allows for the creation of reformatted images in any desired plane after the scan is completed.[19]

Conventional CT is superior to both conventional radiographs and MR imaging for demonstrating bony detail, and is also highly sensitive for detecting even small amounts of calcium hydroxyapatite within the cuff tendons (calcific tendinitis).

Because the soft tissues of the shoulder are otherwise poorly evaluated with conventional CT, CT arthrography has been used as an alternative to MR or

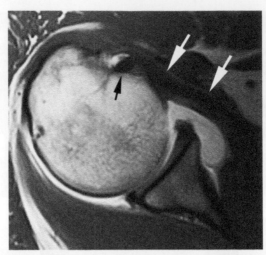

Fig. 9. Axial T1-weighted image (MR arthrogram) demonstrates the subscapularis tendon (*white arrows*) inserting on the lesser tubercle and the long-head biceps tendon within the bicipital groove (*smaller black arrow*).

ultrasonography for imaging the cuff.[20,21] The patient is scanned immediately following the intra-articular injection of 10 to 15 mL of iodinated contrast under fluoroscopic guidance. Using this technique, partial-thickness articular surface and full-thickness cuff tears may be demonstrated along with a detailed depiction of the labrum and articular cartilage (**Fig. 12**).[19] Disadvantages include its poorer overall soft-tissue contrast relative to MR imaging, an inability to demonstrate partial-thickness bursal surface cuff tears, and the need for ionizing radiation.

Magnetic Resonance Imaging

MR imaging has long been considered the premier imaging modality for evaluating internal derangement of the shoulder because it allows for a comprehensive assessment of the entire joint with superb demonstration of bone and soft-tissue abnormality.

Limitations of MR imaging include its relatively long scan times, which may lead to patient motion and associated image degradation. In addition, some patients are unable to undergo an MR scan because of an implanted device considered unsafe in a magnetic field such as a cardiac pacemaker, or because of severe claustrophobia.

Scanning is performed with the patient supine with a surface coil placed over the affected shoulder. The arm is held at the side in external rotation so that the bicipital groove is directed anteriorly. MR arthrography is performed after the intra-articular injection of 12 to 15 mL of a dilute gadolinium solution (typically a 1:200 mix of gadolinium/saline, an off-label use). The resulting joint distention allows for excellent depiction of intra-articular structures.

The arm may also be placed in abduction and external rotation (ABER position), by placing the patient's hand behind the head and repositioning the surface coil over the axilla. This position has been shown to better demonstrate partial thickness under surface tears involving the supraspinatus and infraspinatus tendons as well as tears of the anterior inferior labrum, especially when performed during MR arthrography (**Fig. 13**).[22–24]

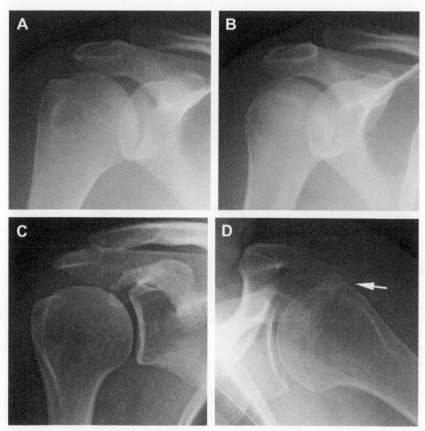

Fig. 10. Radiographic views. (*A*) Anteroposterior (AP)-external rotation. Note the greater tubercle in profile. (*B*) AP-internal rotation. Note the smooth rounded contour of the humeral head. (*C*) Grashey projection. The glenohumeral joint appears more "open". (*D*) Active abduction view. Note the narrowing of the humeral-acromial distance (*arrow*) in this patient with a rotator cuff tear (normal >2 mm).

Shoulder MR imaging protocols vary by institution and depend greatly on the type of scanner being used.

ROTATOR CUFF PATHOLOGY
General Principles

The tendons of the rotator cuff are susceptible to the same pathologic processes as those found elsewhere in the body even though their anatomic positions result in unique physiologic stresses. Tendon failure is typically multifactorial.[25] Advancing age leads to decreased tendon cellularity and vascularity, thinning and disorientation of collagen fibers, and a mixture of myxoid and hyaline degeneration. These changes combined with chronic activity-related microdamage or a single traumatic event may result in tendon failure.[26]

Tendinosis
As a tendon degenerates it typically becomes thickened and demonstrates abnormal signal intensity within its substance on MR imaging related to the myxoid degeneration, chondroid metaplasia, and disoriented collagen fibers.[27]

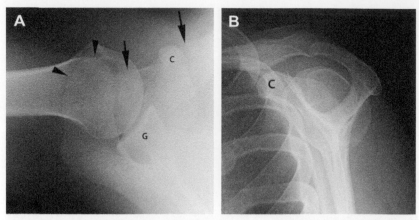

Fig. 11. Radiographic views. (*A*) Axillary view reveals the relationship of the humeral head to the glenoid (G) as well as the coracoid (C), acromion (*arrowheads*), and distal clavicle (*arrows*). (*B*) Outlet view shows the humeral head centered on the glenoid, the coracoid process (C) anteriorly, and the acromioclavicular joint in profile.

Partial-thickness tear

With progressive degeneration and microtrauma, collagen fibers are disrupted, resulting in partial-thickness tearing of the tendon. In a rotator cuff tendon, a partial-thickness tear may involve its articular surface or bursal surface, or may lie entirely within the substance of the tendon without communication with a surface (interstitial tear).

Full-thickness tear

Complete disruption of tendon fibers may occur in a portion of the tendon or may involve the entire tendon as well as others in the cuff ("massive" cuff tear).[28] Varying

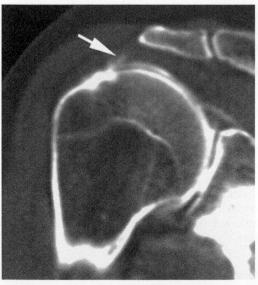

Fig. 12. CT arthrogram. Oblique coronal reconstructed image from a CT arthrogram reveals contrast extending into a small partial-thickness tear of the supraspinatus tendon (*arrow*).

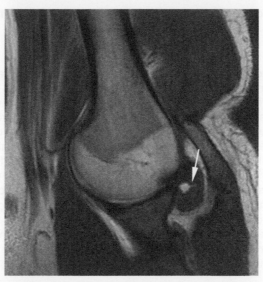

Fig. 13. ABER position. Oblique axial T1-weighted image obtained with the arm abducted and externally rotated (ABER position) demonstrates a small, slit-like partial-thickness tear along the undersurface of the infraspinatus tendon (*arrow*).

degrees of tendon retraction occur, and if the tear is chronic, the affected muscle may undergo significant fatty atrophy.

ROTATOR CUFF IMPINGEMENT

Rotator cuff pathology is commonly related to an impingement syndrome.[2,29,30] Extrinsic impingement results from mechanical impingement of a tendon by an adjacent structure such as the acromion (supraspinatus) or coracoid (subscapularis). This anomaly may occur in a primary form, resulting from abnormal morphology of that structure, or may be secondary to underlying instability of the joint. Internal impingement refers to a syndrome whereby the posterior fibers of the supraspinatus tendon and anterior fibers the infraspinatus tendon are impinged between the greater tuberosity and posterior-superior glenoid when the arm is brought into abduction and external rotation, as with throwing and other overhead athletic activities.

Each of these impingement syndromes affects particular tendons and results in a typical constellation of MR imaging findings.

External Impingement: Supraspinatus

Impingement of the supraspinatus tendon at the level of the coracoacromial arch (anatomic outlet) of the shoulder may be related to the morphology of the acromion, spurring along the undersurface of the anterior acromion and/or acromioclavicular joint or thickening of the coracoacromial ligament.[31] Neer[32] emphasized the importance of the anterior acromion in this process and divided it into 3 stages: (1) acute subacromial bursitis, (2) tendinopathy and partial tearing of the supraspinatus, and (3) progression to a full-thickness tear of the tendon. Bigliani and colleagues[33] described 3 types of acromial morphology: Type 1, flat; Type 2, gentle curve, paralleling the contour of the humeral head; Type 3, a hooked configuration along its undersurface. Bigliani reported a higher incidence of cuff tears in those patients with the

Type 3 configuration. Given these findings, anterior acromioplasty is commonly performed in patients with symptoms of external impingement.

Imaging findings

Radiography Radiographs are helpful for identifying osseous features that might lead to the development of anterior impingement symptoms. Acromial morphology and undersurface spurring can be assessed on outlet view or Stryker notch views of the shoulder, whereas lateral downsloping of the acromion, degenerative changes of the acromioclavicular joint, and the width of the humeral-acromial distance are best seen on frontal views (**Fig. 14**). Cortical irregularity and subcortical lucencies in the greater tuberosity have been described in patients with rotator cuff abnormality, but are nonspecific.[13,34] A persistent os acromiale, whereby it remains unfused in a patient older than 25 years, may be a source of pain, and is demonstrated best on an axillary view. A chronic full-thickness tear may be suspected on radiographs when the humeral-acromial distance is narrowed (less than 6 mm on an AP view or less than 2 mm on an active abduction view) (see **Figs. 10** and **14**),[14] and may be diagnosed on a shoulder arthrogram when contrast extravasates from the joint into the subacromial/subdeltoid bursa.[13]

MR imaging When viewing an MR examination of the shoulder, the same osseous structures assessed on radiographs should be evaluated. Acromial morphology is best assessed on oblique sagittal imaging, as is subacromial or subclavicular spurring (**Fig. 15**). Lateral downsloping of the acromion and the degree of acromioclavicular joint degeneration is well demonstrated on oblique coronal images. Mass effect on the underlying supraspinatus tendon should be commented on, but a diagnosis of impingement syndrome is based on clinical symptoms, not imaging findings.

The spectrum of supraspinatus tendon abnormality ranges from tendinopathy (often with associated subacromial/subdeltoid bursitis) to complete tear. With MR imaging, tendinopathy is diagnosed when tendon thickening and intermediate signal intensity is identified on T1 or proton-density images and then becomes less apparent on more heavily T2-weighted images (**Fig. 16**).[27] Partial-thickness tears most commonly

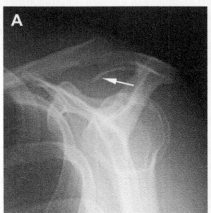
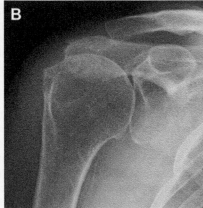

Fig. 14. Radiographic findings. (*A*) Outlet radiograph demonstrates a prominent spur arising from the anterior acromion (*arrow*). (*B*) AP radiograph shows marked narrowing of the humeral-acromial distance compatible with a chronic rotator cuff tear (same patient as in **Fig. 19**B, C).

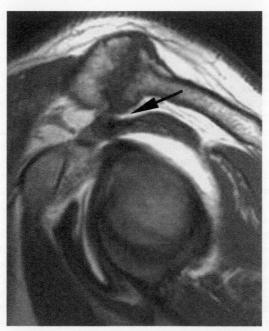

Fig. 15. Acromioclavicular joint degeneration. Oblique sagittal T1-weighted image (MR arthrogram) reveals marked degenerative arthropathy of the acromioclavicular joint with prominent undersurface spurs producing mass effect on the adjacent supraspinatus tendon (*arrow*).

involve the articular surface of the tendon and are diagnosed when focal, fluid-intensity signal is identified extending through a portion of the tendon's substance on T2-weighted images.

A specific type of partial-thickness tear involving the articular surface of the supraspinatus tendon is known as a "rim rent" or PASTA (Partial Articular Supraspinatus Tendon Avulsion) tear.[35,36] These tears are probably related to tensile forces and

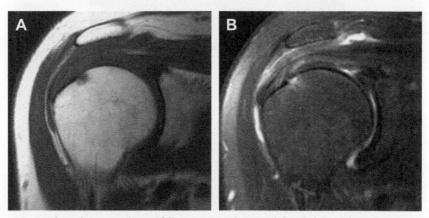

Fig. 16. Tendon degeneration. Oblique coronal T1-weighted (*A*) and T2-weighted (*B*) images show a thickened supraspinatus tendon that demonstrates heterogeneous signal intensity, compatible with degenerative tendinosis.

are often small, involving only a few undersurface fibers. As such, these are easy to overlook on MR imaging. To avoid this error, assessment of the supraspinatus tendon should start at the level of its far anterior margin, which is seen on the oblique coronal image at the level of the biceps tendon as it enters the bicipital groove (**Fig. 17**).

Partial-thickness tears involving the bursal surface of the tendon demonstrate similar findings, but are more difficult to diagnose unless there is fluid within the bursa (**Fig. 18**). Intramuscular cysts may be associated with a partial-thickness tear and prompt a search for a subtle cuff tear.[37]

An interstitial tear is diagnosed when T2-weighted images reveal fluid-like signal within the substance of the tendon that does not extend to its bursal or articular surfaces (see **Fig. 18**). Identifying an interstitial tear on MR imaging is important because it will not be evident at arthroscopy, so if the surgeon is made aware of its presence, that portion of the tendon can be probed, "unroofed" and repaired.

A full-thickness tear is identified when fluid signal intensity (or gadolinium, in the case of an MR arthrogram) extends through the entire substance of the tendon (**Fig. 19**). These tears may be small, involving only a portion of the supraspinatus tendon, or may be "massive" (measuring at least 5 cm in length, often involving the entire supraspinatus and infraspinatus tendons; see **Fig. 19**).[28] Important features of a full-thickness tear that should be assessed on MR images are: (1) the size of the tear in 2 planes, (2) the degree of retraction of the torn margin of the tendon, (3) the quality of the tendon tissue at its torn margins, and (4) the amount of associated fatty atrophy within the cuff muscles, because this has been shown to be associated with poor outcomes after surgical repair.[38,39]

External Impingement: Subscapularis

Impingement of the distal subscapularis tendon between the lesser tuberosity of the humerus and coracoid process, usually with internal rotation of the shoulder, has been termed subcoracoid impingement. Anything that narrows the coracohumeral distance such as congenital or posttraumatic deformity of the coracoid may produce

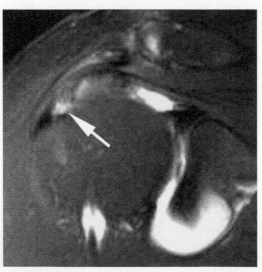

Fig. 17. Partial-thickness tear. Oblique coronal T2-weighted image (MR arthrogram) demonstrates a small partial-thickness undersurface tear involving the distal supraspinatus tendon (*arrow*).

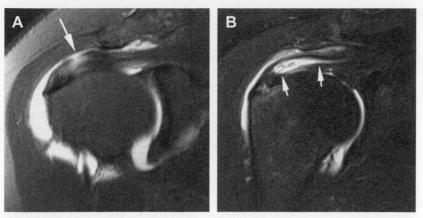

Fig. 18. Partial-thickness tears. (*A*) Oblique coronal T2-weighted image (MR arthrogram) displays a small partial-thickness tear involving the bursal surface of the supraspinatus tendon (*arrow*). (*B*) Oblique coronal T2-weighted image reveals a large interstitial tear causing delamination of the supraspinatus tendon (*arrows*).

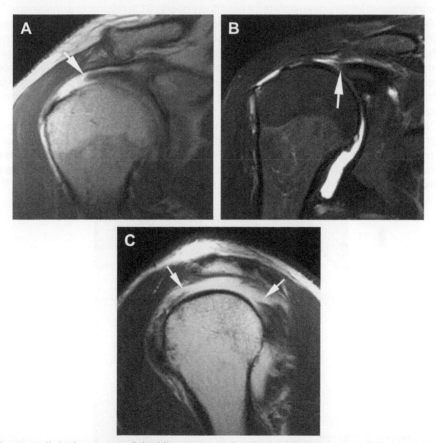

Fig. 19. Full-thickness tears. (*A*) Oblique T1-weighted image (MR arthrogram) demonstrates a full-thickness tear of the supraspinatus tendon with mild retraction of the torn fibers (*arrow*). (*B*) Oblique coronal T2-weighted image (MR arthrogram) in a different patient shows a full-thickness tear with more prominent retraction (*arrow*), and a corresponding oblique sagittal T1-weighted image (*C*) reveals that the tear (between the *arrows*) involves both the supraspinatus and infraspinatus tendons.

symptoms. Other potential causes include anterior joint laxity or insufficiency of the anterosuperior capsule-ligamentous structures in the rotator cuff interval.[40–42] Tears of the subscapularis often occur in conjunction with supraspinatus abnormality, and if missed may result in failed rotator cuff surgery.[2]

Lo and Burkhart[43] described a "roller-wringer" effect of the impingement between the coracoid and lesser tuberosity with internal rotation, leading to undersurface tears of the subscapularis tendon from excessive tensile forces (tensile undersurface fiber failure, ie, TUFF).

Imaging findings

Radiography Conventional radiographs are usually unrevealing in these patients, although anterior subluxation of the humeral head may be seen on an axillary view.

MR imaging Identification of subscapularis abnormality on MR imaging can be challenging. Although one group reported sensitivity of 91% and specificity of 86% for diagnosing these tears with MR arthrography,[44] another retrospective study looking at conventional MR imaging reported a sensitivity of only 31% relative to arthroscopy.[45]

The subscapularis tendon is best evaluated on axial images. Care should be taken to not mistake its normal multipennate structure for longitudinal tearing. As with the other cuff tendons, abnormalities range from tendinopathy (thickening with heterogeneous signal on MR images) to partial tears, usually along the distal articular surface (areas of focal fiber disruption with fluid equivalent signal), to complete disruption with retraction.[42] These distal tears often result in instability and abnormality of the long head of the biceps tendon (**Fig. 20**).

Numerous investigators have attempted to correlate measurements of the coracohumeral distance on cross-sectional imaging studies with symptoms of subcoracoid impingement, but the results have been mixed, primarily because the width of this space is highly dependent on patient positioning, and it is not practical to scan every patient in internal rotation given that this is an uncommon cause of shoulder pain.[46]

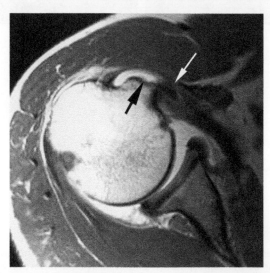

Fig. 20. Subscapularis tear. Axial T1-weighted image (MR arthrogram) reveals partial tearing of the subscapularis tendon from its distal attachment on the lesser tubercle (*black arrow*), allowing the biceps tendon to dislocate out of the bicipital groove into the substance of the tendon (*white arrow*).

External Impingement: Combined Lesions

Combined injuries involving the supraspinatus and subscapularis tendons, are common, and often extend to involve the structures of the rotator cuff interval.[41,47–49]

The exact pathogenesis of these injuries is uncertain, but the initial injury may involve tearing of the biceps "sling", due to a fall on an outstretched arm or repetitive biceps contraction during the deceleration phase of throwing. This rotator interval injury allows subluxation of the biceps tendon at the level of the proximal bicipital groove, often in an anteromedial direction, and development of tears along the superior margin of the subscapularis tendon or anterior margin of the supraspinatus tendon. Over time, these injuries may result in excessive anterior-superior translation of the humeral head with associated impingement against the anterior-superior glenoid on flexion and internal rotation of the arm (as occurs during the follow-through phase of throwing). This phenomenon is termed anterosuperior impingement.[50,51]

MR imaging

Conventional radiographs are often unrevealing in these patients. Similarly, the components of the biceps sling are very difficult, if not impossible, to assess on conventional MR images, and MR arthrography has been advocated in these patients for improved diagnosis.[12,52]

Most often, the tears of the subscapularis and supraspinatus tendons involve the articular surface fibers of their margins that border the rotator cuff interval, and are recognized by fluid or intra-articular contrast extending between the tendon and bone. Subluxation of the biceps tendon is best assessed on axial images, although associated tendinopathy or partial tearing often requires evaluation of the tendon in all 3 planes owing to its curvilinear course as it extends over the humeral head. The coracohumeral and superior glenohumeral ligaments (biceps sling) are best evaluated in the oblique sagittal projection, and when injured appear ill-defined or disrupted, often with associated synovial irregularity (synovitis) (**Fig. 21**).

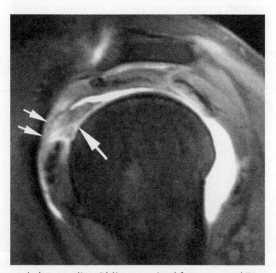

Fig. 21. Rotator interval abnormality. Oblique sagittal fat-saturated T1-weighted image (MR arthrogram) demonstrates partial tearing of a thickened biceps tendon (*large arrow*) and disruption of the biceps pulley structures (*small arrows*).

Internal Impingement: Infraspinatus and Posterior Supraspinatus

With abduction and external rotation of the shoulder during throwing and other over-head motions, the greater tuberosity of the humerus contacts the posterior-superior glenoid. This phenomenon is a normal one that is usually asymptomatic, but in some athletes this impingement of the posterior cuff tendons (anterior infraspinatus and posterior supraspinatus) against the posterior-superior portion of the glenoid may produce pain known as internal or posterior-superior impingement.[53–55]

The etiology of this syndrome is probably multifactorial. Some suggest that anterior capsular laxity and/or microinstability in throwing athletes may permit excessive external rotation that contributes to symptomatic impingement.[56] Others postulate that a pathologic cascade begins with tightening of the posterior capsule and the posterior band of the inferior glenohumeral ligament, resulting in a loss of internal rotation and posterior-superior shift of the humeral axis of rotation relative to the glenoid (termed glenohumeral internal rotation deficit, ie, GIRD).[57]

Regardless of cause, this syndrome results in a constellation of findings including: (1) partial-thickness undersurface tears involving the posterior supraspinatus and anterior infraspinatus tendons, (2) posterior-superior labral fraying/tearing, (3) cystic changes in the posterior aspect of the greater tuberosity, and (4) subchondral sclerosis in the posterior-superior glenoid.[2,58–61]

Imaging findings

Radiography Radiographs are often unrevealing in these patients, although certain findings may be present. Calcification along the posterior joint capsule (Bennett lesion), sclerosis or subchondral lucencies in the greater tuberosity, and rounding of the posterior margin of the glenoid (on axillary view) have been described.[53]

MR imaging Undersurface tears involving the supraspinatus and infraspinatus tendons that occur with posterior-superior impingement are often subtle and difficult to detect with conventional MR imaging. As a result, MR arthrography has been rec-ommended in these patients (**Fig. 22**). Scanning with the patient in the ABER position has also been advocated because this allows for better depiction of the articular surface of the cuff than does scanning with the arm at the side.[22,62,63] Associated

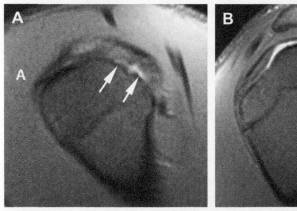

Fig. 22. Internal impingement. (*A*) Oblique sagittal fat-saturated T1-weighted image in a college baseball pitcher shows an undersurface tear of the infraspinatus tendon (*arrows*; A = anterior). (*B*) Oblique coronal fat-saturated T1-weighted image in the same patient reveals an associated tear of the posterior superior labrum (*arrow*).

cystic foci within the greater tuberosity or posterior-superior glenoid are best seen on fat-saturated T2-weighted images. The posterior-superior labrum should also be scrutinized for abnormality, and is best demonstrated on oblique coronal images (see **Fig. 22**). The identification of one or more of these findings in an overhead athlete should suggest the possibility of posterior-superior impingement, but must be viewed in concert with the clinical examination because these findings may be seen in asymptomatic throwers.

MISCELLANEOUS DISORDERS OF THE ROTATOR CUFF
Adhesive Capsulitis

Adhesive capsulitis, also known as frozen shoulder, is a disorder of uncertain etiology that begins with the spontaneous onset of often severe shoulder pain and decreased range of motion. The underlying pathology involves fibroblastic proliferation within the joint capsule resulting in capsular thickening and contraction. It more commonly affects diabetic patients, females, and patients who have sustained prior trauma, but may arise without an identifiable cause.[64,65]

An initial phase of increasing pain and decreasing range of motion may progress over several months. The pain and limited motion will often plateau in a second phase that lasts several more months, and then spontaneously regress (third phase) over another 1 to 2 years.[64] Steroid injections and physical therapy may help to shorten the duration of symptoms. Although diagnosis is most commonly based on clinical findings, it can be difficult because adhesive capsulitis may mimic other types of intra-articular pathology.

Imaging findings
Radiography Conventional radiographs are typically unrevealing, but conventional arthrographic findings include an increased resistance to injection at a low volume, a serrated appearance of the joint capsule, and a loss or shrinkage of capsular recesses.[66]

MR imaging Several MR imaging findings have been reported in patients with adhesive capsulitis including thickening of the coracohumeral ligament,[67,68] infiltration of the retrocoracoid fat by intermediate signal intensity tissue on T1-weighted images,[67-69] and capsular thickening in the axillary pouch,[70] although the reliability of this latter finding has been questioned (**Fig. 23**). Because the capsule may appear thickened on conventional MR images owing to a lack of joint distention, MR arthrography has been recommended for better evaluation. If intravenous gadolinium is used, pronounced capsular thickening and enhancement may be seen in the active phases of the disease.[71]

Calcium Hydroxyapatite Deposition Disease

Calcium hydroxyapatite deposition disease (HADD), also known as calcific tendinitis, may occur anywhere in the body but most commonly affects the shoulder, and most often involves the supraspinatus tendon.[72] Although it begins with a "silent" phase in which clinical symptoms are mild or nonexistent, its later phases are marked by pronounced shoulder pain when the associated calcium salts rupture into the tendon and/or adjacent bursa.[73]

Imaging findings
Radiography Conventional radiographs reveal one or more foci of amorphous calcification within the affected tendon (**Fig. 24**). The calcification may increase in size or spontaneously disappear over time. With bursal involvement, a thin margin of calcium

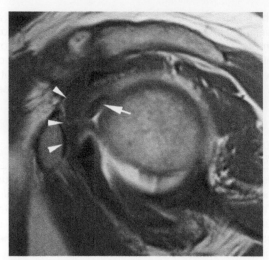

Fig. 23. Adhesive capsulitis. Oblique sagittal T1-weighted image (MR arthrogram) demonstrates marked thickening of the anterior capsular structures and intermediate-signal-intensity tissue infiltrating the retrocoracoid fat (*arrowheads*), a finding often seen in patients with adhesive capsulitis (*arrow* indicates biceps tendon).

outlining the bursa may be seen. Cortical erosion can occur at the insertion of an involved tendon, sometimes mimicking a surface neoplasm.[66,74]

CT CT is more sensitive than radiographs for detecting and/or defining the appearance and location of the calcific deposits.[66,72]

MR imaging Small foci of calcification may be easily missed on MR images because the low signal intensity of the calcium blends with the low-signal tendon fibers on all pulse sequences. Gradient-echo sequences are helpful in this regard given the "blooming" artifact that accompanies the calcification (see **Fig. 24**). Because of the

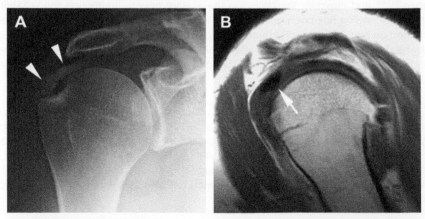

Fig. 24. Calcific tendinitis. (*A*) AP radiograph demonstrates prominent, amorphous calcification in the supraspinatus tendon (*arrowheads*) compatible with hydroxyapatite deposition disease (calcific tendinitis). (*B*) Oblique sagittal T1-weighted image in the same patient reveals a large focus of low-signal-intensity calcium causing focal thickening of the supraspinatus tendon (*arrow*).

superb soft tissue contrast of MR imaging, the inflammatory changes accompanying HADD may mimic an infectious or neoplastic process, and correlation with radiographs is essential to avoid misdiagnosis.[75]

Neurologic Conditions

Denervation

Injury or compression of the suprascapular nerve will result in pathologic changes in the supraspinatus and/or infraspinatus muscles. Similarly, entrapment or injury of the axillary nerve will affect the teres minor and/or deltoid muscles.[76] Although these conditions are typically evident on electromyography, this may not be obtained because of a confusing clinical picture.

MR imaging findings MR imaging is very useful in these patients because of its ability to demonstrate abnormal signal intensity within denervated muscles in the early phases of the process. With acute to subacute denervation (days to weeks), increased "edema-like" signal intensity is seen within the affected muscles that is thought to occur as a result of increased capillary blood volume (**Fig. 25**).[77] If the muscle is reinnervated at this point, the signal will fade over time, but if not, fatty infiltration will become more evident over the course of months, as evidenced by increasing high-signal tissue within the muscles that is irreversible. When these findings are observed within the muscles supplied by a common nerve, denervation injury should be suspected and the course of the nerve scrutinized for evidence of injury or compressing mass.

Parsonage-Turner syndrome

Also known as acute brachial neuritis or neuralgic amyotrophy, this idiopathic syndrome begins with an abrupt onset of shoulder pain that often mimics other causes of intra-articular abnormality. This syndrome is usually a self-limited disease that resolves over the course of several months, but may mimic other types of shoulder abnormality and is usually a diagnosis of exclusion.

MR imaging findings The diagnosis of Parsonage-Turner syndrome may be suggested when the MR findings of denervation described in the prior section are seen

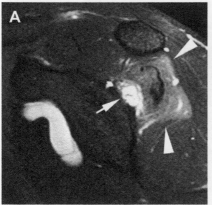
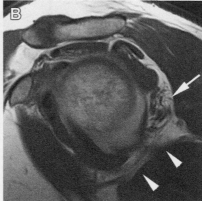

Fig. 25. Denervation. (*A*) Oblique sagittal T2-weighted image (MR arthrogram) shows diffusely increased signal within the infraspinatus muscle (*arrowheads*) secondary to denervation from compression of the suprascapular nerve by posterior paralabral cysts (*arrow*). (*B*) Oblique sagittal T1-weighted image in a different patient shows prominent fatty atrophy of the teres minor muscle (*arrow*) without evidence of abnormality along the course of the axillary nerve in the quadrilateral space (*arrowheads*). This finding is often of an idiopathic nature.

within periscapular muscles, and should be especially considered when muscles innervated by both the suprascapular and axillary nerves are involved.[76,78,79] MR imaging is also useful for eliminating other cases of shoulder pain that may result in a similar clinical picture.

POSTOPERATIVE ROTATOR CUFF

Treatment decisions in a patient with rotator cuff abnormality will depend on several factors including the patient's age, activity level, the size of tear, degree of retraction, and amount of fatty atrophy in the cuff muscles. Most cuff repairs are performed arthroscopically and are often combined with an arthroscopic acromioplasty.

Imaging Findings

Radiography
Conventional radiographs should be the first study obtained, and are useful for assessing morphology of the acromion and/or distal clavicle and whether there are any metallic fixation devices that may affect cross-sectional imaging.[80,81]

CT
Standard CT imaging can be used to evaluate the shoulder, in many cases even if metallic fixation devices have been used, because newer scanning techniques significantly reduce metal-related artifacts. CT arthrography is the study of choice in those patients in whom MR imaging is not possible because of metal-related artifacts or a contraindication to MR imaging such as a cardiac pacemaker.[80]

MR imaging
MR imaging of the shoulder after acromioplasty and/or cuff repair can be challenging for several reasons, including distortion of normal anatomy, the presence of postoperative scar, and metal-related artifacts from fixation hardware or prior burring or drilling of bone (**Fig. 26**).

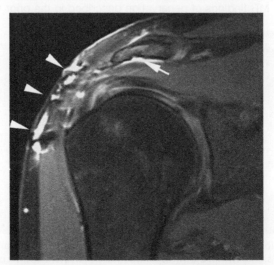

Fig. 26. Postoperative shoulder. Oblique coronal fat-saturated T2-weighted image in a patient after acromioplasty shows extensive artifacts within the soft tissues related to microscopic metallic debris (*arrowheads*) as well as a small amount of fluid within the subacromial bursa outlining a tapered and irregular undersurface of the acromion (*arrow*).

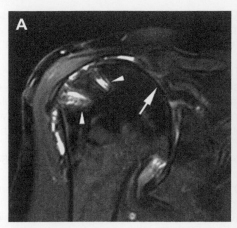
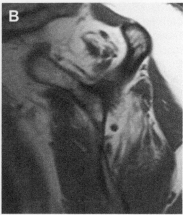

Fig. 27. Recurrent rotator cuff tear. (A) Oblique coronal fat-saturated T2-weighted image demonstrates a massive, recurrent tear of the cuff with marked retraction (arrow). Note also the residua of prior fixation devices in the greater tuberosity (arrowheads). (B) Oblique sagittal T1-weighted image in the same patient reveals severe fatty atrophy of the supraspinatus and infraspinatus muscles.

After acromioplasty, morphology of the acromion is variable, but not predictive of clinical symptoms or probability of developing a recurrent cuff tear.[82] Edema-like signal intensity may persist within the humeral head marrow for months or years after repair, especially if transosseous sutures have been used.[80]

Relatively few patients will demonstrate a normal-appearing rotator cuff after repair.[83] Repairs are often not watertight, so partial or full-thickness "tears" are commonly seen in asymptomatic patients, although it has been shown that cuff defects larger than 1 cm are more often associated with symptoms (**Fig. 27**).[84] As such, imaging findings must be closely correlated with clinical symptoms in these patients. Detection of fatty atrophy of the cuff musculature is important if a repair is contemplated after a postoperative failure (see **Fig. 27**). MR imaging also allows for detection of other causes of postoperative pain such as denervation or infection.

ACKNOWLEDGMENT

Special thanks to Phil Cohen for providing the color diagrams.

REFERENCES

1. Clark JM, Harryman H. Tendons, ligaments, and capsule of the rotator cuff: gross and microscopic anatomy. J Bone Joint Surg Am 1992;74:713–25.
2. Roh MS, Wang VM, April EW, et al. Anterior and posterior musculotendinous anatomy of the supraspinatus. J Shoulder Elbow Surg 2000;9:436–40.
3. Opsha O, Malik A, Baltazar R, et al. MRI of the rotator cuff and internal derangement. Eur J Radiol 2008;68:36–56.
4. MacDonald K, Bridger J, Cash C, et al. Transverse humeral ligament: does it exist? Clin Anat 2007;20:663–7.
5. Gleason PD, Beall DP, Sanders TG, et al. The transverse humeral ligament: a separate anatomical structure or a continuation of the osseous attachment of the rotator cuff? Am J Sports Med 2006;34(1):72–7.

6. Curtis AS, Burbank KM, Tierney DO, et al. The insertional footprint of the rotator cuff: an anatomic study. Arthroscopy 2006;22:603–9.
7. Benjamin M, Evans EJ, Copp L. The histology of tendon attachments to bone in man. J Anat 1986;149:89–100.
8. Burkhart SS, Esch JC, Jolson RS. The rotator crescent and rotator cable: an anatomic description of the shoulder's "suspension bridge". Arthroscopy 1993;9:611–6.
9. Sheah K, Bredella MA, Warner JJ, et al. Transverse thickening along the articular surface of the rotator cuff consistent with the rotator cable: identification with MR arthrography and relevance in rotator cuff evaluation. AJR Am J Roentgenol 2009;193:679–86.
10. Krief OP. MRI of the rotator interval capsule. AJR Am J Roentgenol 2005;184:1490–4.
11. Hunt SA, Kwon YW, Zuckerman JD. The rotator interval: anatomy, pathology and strategies for treatment. J Am Acad Orthop Surg 2007;15:218–27.
12. Petchprapa CN, Beltran LS, Jazrawi LM, et al. The rotator interval: a review of anatomy, function, and normal and abnormal MRI appearance. AJR Am J Roentgenol 2010;195:567–76.
13. Huang BK, Hughes TH. Imaging of the rotator cuff. Sports Med Arthrosc 2011;19:279–99.
14. Moosikasuwan JB, Miller TT, Burke BJ. Rotator cuff tears: clinical radiographic and US findings. Radiographics 2005;25:1591–607.
15. Teefey SA, Rubin DA, Middleton WD, et al. Detection and quantification of rotator cuff tears. J Bone Joint Surg AM 2004;86:708–16.
16. Rutten MJ, Spaargaren GJ, van Loon T, et al. Detection of rotator cuff tears: the value of MRI following ultrasound. Eur Radiol 2010;20:450–7.
17. Vlychou M, Dailiana Z, Fotiodou A, et al. Symptomatic partial rotator cuff tears: diagnostic performance of ultrasound and magnetic resonance imaging with surgical correlation. Acta Radiol 2009;50:101–5.
18. Sipola P, Niemitukia L, Kroger H, et al. Detection and quantification of rotator cuff tears with ultrasonography and magnetic resonance imaging: a prospective study in 77 consecutive patients with a surgical reference. Ultrasound Med Biol 2010;36:1981–9.
19. Fritz J, Fishman EK, Small KM, et al. MDCT arthrography of the shoulder with datasets of isotropic resolution: indications, technique, and applications. AJR Am J Roentgenol 2012;198:635–46.
20. DeFilippo M, Bertellini A, Sverzellati N, et al. Multidetector computed tomography arthrography of the shoulder: diagnostic accuracy and indications. Acta Radiol 2008;49:540–9.
21. Oh JH, Kim JY, Choi JA, et al. Effectiveness of multidetector computed tomography arthrography for the diagnosis of shoulder pathology: comparison with magnetic resonance imaging with arthroscopic correlation. J Shoulder Elbow Surg 2010;19:14–20.
22. Jung JY, Jee WH, Chun HJ, et al. Magnetic resonance arthrography including ABER view in diagnosing partial-thickness tears of the rotator cuff: accuracy, and inter- and intra-observer agreements. Acta Radiol 2010;51:194–201.
23. Roger B, Skaf A, Hooper AW, et al. Imaging findings in the dominant shoulder of throwing athletes: comparison of radiography, arthrography, CT arthrography and MR arthrography with arthroscopic correlation. AJR Am J Roentgenol 1999;172:1371–80.
24. Cvitanic O, Tirman PF, Fell JF, et al. Using abduction and external rotation of the shoulder to increase the sensitivity of MR arthrography in revealing tears of the anterior glenoid labrum. AJR Am J Roentgenol 1997;169:837–44.

25. Lewis JS. Rotator cuff tendinopathy. Br J Sports Med 2009;43:236–41.
26. Nho SJ, Yadav H, Shindle MK, et al. Rotator cuff degeneration: etiology and pathogenesis. Am J Sports Med 2008;36:987–93.
27. Buck FM, Grehn H, Hilbe M, et al. Magnetic resonance histologic correlation in rotator cuff tendons. J Magn Reson Imaging 2010;32:165–72.
28. Bedi A, Dines J, Warren RF, et al. Massive tears of the rotator cuff. J Bone Joint Surg Am 2010;92:1894–908.
29. Ouellett H, Kassarjian A, Tretreault P, et al. Imaging of the overhead throwing athlete. Semin Musculoskelet Radiol 2005;9:316–33.
30. Anderson MW, Alford BA. Overhead throwing injuries of the shoulder and elbow. Radiol Clin North Am 2010;48:1137–54.
31. Harrison AK, Flatow EL. Subacromial impingement syndrome. J Am Acad Orthop Surg 2011;19:701–8.
32. Neer CS II. Anterior acromioplasty for the chronic impingement syndrome in the shoulder: a preliminary report. J Bone Joint Surg Am 1972;54:41–50.
33. Bigliani LU, Morrison DS, April EW. The morphology of the acromion and its relationship to rotator cuff tears. Orthop Trans 1986;10:216.
34. Gazzola S, Bleakney RR. Current imaging of the rotator cuff. Sports Med Arthrosc 2011;19:300–9.
35. Vinson EN, Helms CA, Higgins LD. Rim-rent tear of the rotator cuff: a common and easily overlooked partial tear. AJR Am J Roentgenol 2007;189:943–6.
36. Tuite MJ, Turnbull JR, Orwin JF. Anterior versus posterior and rim-rent rotator cuff tears: prevalence and MR sensitivity. Skeletal Radiol 1998;27:237–43.
37. Manvar AM, Kamireddi A, Bhalani SM, et al. Clinical significance of intramuscular cysts in the rotator cuff and their relationship to full- and partial-thickness rotator cuff tears. AJR Am J Roentgenol 2009;192:719–24.
38. Thomazeau H, Boukobza E, Morcet N, et al. Prediction of rotator cuff repair results by magnetic resonance imaging. Clin Orthop 1997;344:275–83.
39. Goutallier D, Postel JM, Gleyze P, et al. Influence of cuff muscle fatty degeneration on anatomic and functional outcomes after simple suture of full-thickness tears. J Shoulder Elbow Surg 2003;12(6):550–4.
40. Garofalo R, Conti M, Massazza G, et al. Subcoracoid impingement syndrome: a painful shoulder condition related to different pathologic factors. Musculoskelet Surg 2001;95(Suppl 1):S25–9.
41. Morag Y, Jamadar DA, Miller B, et al. The subscapularis: anatomy, injury, and imaging. Skeletal Radiol 2011;40:255–69.
42. Lyons RP, Green A. Subscapularis tendon tears. J Am Acad Orthop Surg 2005; 13:353–63.
43. Lo IK, Burkhart SS. The etiology and assessment of subscapularis tendon tears: a case for subcoracoid impingement, the roller-wringer effect, an tuff lesions of the subscapularis. Arthroscopy 2003;19:1142–50.
44. Pfirmann CS, Zanetti M, Weishaupt D, et al. Subscapularis tendon tears: detection and grading at MR arthrography. Radiology 1999;213:709–14.
45. Tung GA, Yoo DC, Levine SM, et al. Subscapularis tendon tear: primary and associated signs on MRI. J Comput Assist Tomogr 2001;25:417–24.
46. Giaroli EL, Major NM, Lemley DE, et al. Coracohumeral interval imaging in subcoracoid impingement syndrome on MRI. AJR Am J Roentgenol 2006;186: 242–6.
47. Lo IKY, Parten PM, Burkhart SS. Combined sucoracoid and cubacromial impingement in association with anterosuperior rotator cuff tears: an arthroscopic approach. Arthroscopy 2003;19:1068–78.

48. Macmahon PJ, Taylor DH, Duke D, et al. Contribution of full-thickness supraspinatus tendon tears to acquired subcoracoid impingement. Clin Radiol 2007;62: 556–63.
49. Braun S, Horan MP, Elser F, et al. Lesions of the biceps pulley. Am J Sports Med 2011;39:790–5.
50. Habermyer P, Magosch P, Pritsch M, et al. Anterosuperior impingement of the shoulder as a result of pulley lesions: a prospective arthroscopic study. J Shoulder Elbow Surg 2004;13:5–12.
51. Garofalo R, Karlsson J, Nordenson U, et al. Anterior-superior internal impingement of the shoulder: an evidence-based review. Knee Surg Sports Traumatol Arthrosc 2010;18:1688–93.
52. Nakata W, Katou S, Fujita A, et al. Biceps pullet: normal anatomy and associated lesions at MR arthrography. Radiographics 2011;31:791–810.
53. Heyworth BE, Williams RJ. Internal impingement of the shoulder. Am J Sports Med 2009;37:1024.
54. Castagna A, Garofalo R, Cesari E, et al. Posterior superior impingement: an evidence-based review. Br J Sports Med 2010;44:382–8.
55. Kirchhoff C, Imhoff AB. Posterosuperior and anterosuperior impingement of the shoulder in overhead athletes – evolving concepts. Int Orthop 2010;34:1049–58.
56. Paley KJ, Jobe FW, Pink MM, et al. Arthroscopic findings in the overhand throwing athlete: evidence for posterior internal impingement of the rotator cuff. Arthroscopy 2000;16:35–40.
57. Burkhart SS, Morgan CD, Kibler WB. The disabled throwing shoulder: spectrum of pathology. Part I, pathoanatomy and biomechanics. Arthroscopy 2003;19: 404–20.
58. Giaroli EL, Major NM, Higgins LD. MRI of internal impingement of the shoulder. AJR Am J Roentgenol 2005;185:925–9.
59. Kapln LD, McMahon PJ, Towers J, et al. Internal impingement: findings on magnetic resonance imaging and arthroscopic evaluation. Arthroscopy 2004; 20:701–4.
60. Halbrecht JL, Tirman P, Atkin D. Internal impingement of the shoulder: comparison of findings between the throwing and non-throwing shoulders of college baseball players. Arthroscopy 1999;25:253–8.
61. Tuite MJ, Persen BD, Wise SM, et al. Shoulder MR arthrography of the posterior labrocapsular complex in overhead throwers with pathologic internal impingement and internal rotation deficit. Skeletal Radiol 2007;36:495–502.
62. Tirman PF, Bost FW, Garvin GJ, et al. Posterosuperior glenoid impingement of the shoulder: findings at MR imaging and MR arthrography with arthroscopic correlation. Radiology 1994;193:431–6.
63. Tuire MJ. MR imaging of sports injuries to the rotator cuff. Magn Reson Imaging Clin N Am 2003;11:207–19.
64. Zuckerman JD, Rokito A. Frozen shoulder: a consensus definition. J Shoulder Elbow Surg 2011;20:322–5.
65. Hand GC, Athanasou NA, Mattews T, et al. The pathology of frozen shoulder. J Bone Joint Surg Br 2007;89:928–32.
66. Farid N, Bruce D, Chung CB. Miscellaneous conditions of the shoulder: anatomical, clinical, and pictorial review emphasizing potential pitfalls in imaging diagnosis. Eur J Radiol 2008;68:88–105.
67. Lee SY, Park J, Song SW. Correlation of MR arthrographic findings and range of shoulder motions in patients with frozen shoulder. AJR Am J Roentgenol 2012; 198:173–9.

68. Mangiardi B, Pfirmann CW, Gerber C, et al. Frozen shoulder: MR arthrographic findings. Radiology 2004;233:486–92.
69. Kerimoglu U, Aydingoz U, Atay OA, et al. Magnetic resonance imaging of the rotator interval in patients on long-term hemodialysis: correlation with the range of shoulder motions. J Comput Assist Tomogr 2007;31:970–5.
70. Emig EW, Schweitzer ME, Karasick D, et al. Adhesive capsulitis of the shoulder: MR diagnosis. AJR Am J Roentgenol 1995;164:1457–9.
71. Carillon Y, Noel E, Fantino O, et al. Magnetic resonance imaging findings in idio-pathic adhesive capsulitis of the shoulder. Rev Rhum Engl Ed 1999;66:201–6.
72. Garcia GM, McCord GC, Kumar R. Hydroxyapatite crystal deposition disease. Semin Musculoskelet Radiol 2003;7:187–93.
73. Hayes CW, Conway WF. Calcium hydroxyapatite deposition disease. Radio-graphics 1990;10:1031–48.
74. Flemming DJ, Murphey MD, Shekitka KM, et al. Osseous involvement in calcific tendinitis; a retrospective review of 50 cases. AJR Am J Roentgenol 2003;181:965–72.
75. Chung CB, Gentili A, Chew FS. Calcific tendinosis and periarthritis: classic magnetic resonance imaging appearance and associated findings. J Comput Assist Tomogr 2004;28:390–6.
76. Yanny S, Toms AP. MR patterns of denervation around the shoulder. AJR Am J Roentgenol 2010;195:W157–63.
77. Kamath S, Venkatanarasimha N, Walsh MA, et al. MRI appearance of muscle denervation. Skeletal Radiol 2008;37:397–404.
78. Gaskin CM, Helms CA. Parsonage-Turner syndrome: MR imaging findings and clinical information of 27 patients. Radiology 2006;240:501–7.
79. Scalf RE, Wenger DE, Grick MA, et al. MRI findings of 26 patients with Parsonage-Turner syndrome. AJR Am J Roentgenol 2007;189:W39–44.
80. Woertler K. Multimodality imaging of the postoperative shoulder. Eur Radiol 2007;17:3038–55.
81. Mohana-Borges AV, Chung CB, Resnick D. MR imaging an d MR arthrography of the postoperative shoulder: spectrum of normal and abnormal findings. Radio-graphics 2004;24:69–85.
82. Koh KH, Laddha MS, Lim TK, et al. A magnetic resonance imaging study of 100 cases of arthroscopic acromioplasty. Am J Sports Med 2012;40:352–8.
83. Spielmann AL, Foster BB, Kokan P, et al. Shoulder after rotator cuff repair: MR imaging findings in asymptomatic individuals—initial experience. Radiology 1999;213:705–8.
84. Zanetti M, Jost B, Hodler J, et al. MR imaging after rotator cuff repair: full-thickness defect and bursitis-like subacromial abnormalities in asymptomatic subjects. Skeletal Radiol 2000;29:314–9.

Arthroscopic Rotator Cuff Repair
Techniques in 2012

James E. Voos, MD*, Cris D. Barnthouse, MD,
Andrew R. Scott, MD

KEYWORDS

- Rotator cuff, Single-row • Double-row • Transosseous equvialent

KEY POINTS

- Rotator cuff (RTC) repair techniques have evolved over the past 2 decades from open, to miniopen, and now all-arthroscopic repair.
- Partial-thickness tears of the RTC are more common than full-thickness tears and may be a significant source of pain secondary to nonphysiologic tension in the remaining intact fibers.
- When selecting an RTC repair technique, it is important to identify the tear pattern and adhere to the fundamentals of tendon mobilization and footprint preparation.

INTRODUCTION

Multiple studies have documented the transition to arthroscopic techniques as technology and instrumentation have continued to advance. A 2005 survey of 167 orthopedic surgeons found that 62% would repair a mobile 3-cm tear arthroscopically.[1] This was an increase from 2002, when Dunn and colleagues[2] reported 14.5% of surgeons preferred an arthroscopic approach. Colvin and colleagues[3] reported the number of arthroscopic RTC repairs increased by 600% between 1996 and 2006. During the same time interval, open repairs still increased, however, only by 34%. In addition, evolution of arthroscopic techniques has allowed for reproducible repairs of partial-thickness and massive RTC tears.

FUNDAMENTALS

Regardless of the repair configuration used, the fundamentals of RTC repair remain the same. Proper patient positioning, anesthesia, portal placement, visualization, bony footprint preparation, and tendon mobilization allow for a successful outcome. A critical step in RTC repair is recognition of the tear pattern. Once the tear configuration has

The authors have no financial conflicts to disclose.
Orthopaedic and Sports Medicine Clinic of Kansas City, 3651 College Boulevard, Leawood, KS 66211, USA
* Corresponding author.
E-mail address: JVOOS@OSMCKC.COM

been properly identified, the surgeon can select the most appropriate technique to best restore the anatomic footprint and balance force couples of the RTC.

Partial-thickness tears are divided into either articular-sided or bursal-sided tears. Ellman[4] classified partial-thickness tears based on the amount of tendon involved at the footprint insertion: grade I tears involve less than 3 mm of the tendon, grade II tears involve between 3 mm and 6 mm, and grade III tears involve greater than 6 mm of the tendon insertion. Full-thickness RTC tears have classically been divided into 4 categories: crescent-shaped, U-shaped, L-shaped, and massive tears.[5] Several studies have quantified RTC tears based on size and footprint dimensions. RTC tears have been quantified as small, less than 1 cm; medium, 1 cm to 3 cm; large, greater than 3 cm; and massive, greater than 5 cm. In a cadaveric study, Dugas and colleagues[6] reported the mean transverse dimension of the insertion as 14.7 mm. In a more recent study, Mochizuki and colleagues[7] concluded the footprint of the supraspinatus is triangular in shape, with an average maximum medial-to-lateral dimension of 6.9 mm and an average maximum anteroposterior width of 12.6 mm. The infraspinatus has a larger footprint area with a trapezoidal shape. The average maximum medial-to-lateral length is 10.2 mm and average maximum anteroposterior width of 32.7 mm. Finally, Goutallier and colleagues[8] outlined a system to quantify the amount of fatty degeneration in the RTC musculature on preoperative imaging as an important factor contributing to RTC function after repair.

The optimal RTC repair construct has been outlined by several investigators in attempts to restore glenohumeral kinematics.[5,9,10] The goals of RTC repair are to restore footprint anatomy with a biomechanically secure, tension-free construct that promotes biologic healing at the tendon-to-bone interface.

Recent data have raised concern over the high rate of structural failure in the RTC after single-row suture anchor repairs, with recurrent tear rates ranging from 19% to 94% despite good clinical outcomes.[11–16] Additional studies have concluded that patients with a healed RTC repair, with confirmed repair site integrity on postoperative imaging, demonstrate improved strength and functional outcomes when compared with patients with recurrent defects[10,14,15,17–19] Based on these findings, double-row suture anchor and transosseous-equivalent repair techniques were developed in attempts to improve the structural and functional outcomes in patients with symptomatic RTC tears.[9,20]

PARTIAL-THICKNESS ROTATOR CUFF REPAIR

Partial-thickness tears of the RTC are more common than full-thickness tears and may be a significant source of pain secondary to nonphysiologic tension in the remaining intact fibers. Mazzocca and colleagues[21] demonstrated in biomechanical studies that the presence of partial-thickness RTC tears altered strain patterns in the remaining cuff, ultimately resulting in tear propagation. Yamanaka and Matsumato[22] demonstrated partial RTC tears demonstrate no spontaneous healing, and the natural history of such tears seems to be progressive extension of the tear. These biomechanical studies of strain alteration leading to further tendon tearing present a rationale for repair in symptomatic partial-thickness RTC tears.

When attempts at nonsurgical treatment fail to relieve symptoms, surgical treatment may be indicated. Duralde and McClelland[23] found a high percentage of patients with partial-thickness RTC tears treated surgically have associated pathology warranting treatment (**Fig. 1**). Poorer results without correction of concomitant pathologies have been identified.

Multiple techniques have been described for surgical treatment of partial-thickness tears, but these generally fall into 2 categories: (1) arthroscopic RTC débridement and

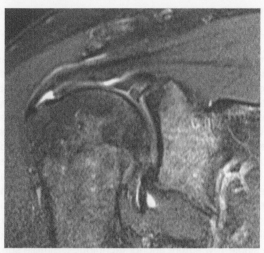

Fig. 1. MRI of a right shoulder with a PASTA RTC tear. There is a concomitant superior labral tear.

(2) repair with or without acromioplasty. There is no high level evidence in the literature to support a specific surgical technique but data suggest repair is usually indicated if bursal-sided and articular tears involve more than 50% of tendon thickness. Débridement is generally used when less than 50% of the RTC is torn.[23-26]

Surgical repair techniques for partial RTC tears include either conversion to a full-thickness tear when the remaining fibers are of poor quality, followed by either a single-row or double-row repair as indicated, or, alternatively, repair of partial articular-sided tendon avulsion (PASTA) tears can be performed with a transtendon technique, restoring the RTC footprint while preserving the intact superficial fibers and maximizing greater tuberosity contact.[23-26] With the transtendon technique, the torn articular-sided fibers are débrided and the exposed bony footprint is prepared. If more than 6 mm to 7 mm of footprint is exposed this suggests 50% or more of the tendon is involved, and a suture anchor is placed percutaneously into the medial aspect of the exposed footprint for repair. A concern for the transtendon approach is overtightening of the bursal fibers, resulting in shoulder stiffness.

Clinical studies have demonstrated favorable results with both techniques. Duralde and McClellan[23] retrospectively reviewed 50 patients treated with arthroscopic transtendinous repair for Ellman grade III articular-sided RTC tears and reported 98% of patients were satisfied with the results of the surgery. Preoperative MRI and magnetic resonance arthrography were accurate in identifying a partial-thickness RTC tear in less than 40% of cases. Strauss and colleagues[26] performed a systematic review of 16 studies on the management of symptomatic partial-thickness RTC tears. The investigators concluded there is no evidence to suggest a difference in outcome for tear completion and repair versus transtendon repair because both methods have been shown to result in successful outcomes. Most recently, Shin performed a prospective, randomized study of 48 patients undergoing either transtendon repair or tear completion and repair.[27] Clinical outcomes significantly improved in both groups at a mean follow-up of 31 months. In addition to decreased pain in the first 3 postoperative months, shoulder function and range of motion recovered faster in the tear completion group. At 6 months' follow up, MRI revealed no retears in the transtendon group and 2 retears in the tear completion group.

FULL-THICKNESS ROTATOR CUFF REPAIR
Single-Row

Single-row suture anchor techniques typically use a linear row of anchors inserted approximately 5 mm lateral to the articular surface.[27] Anchors are ideally placed with a deadman angle, as described by Burkhart and Lo,[5] of less than 45°. Using double-loaded and/or triple-loaded suture anchor reduces the load at the suture-tendon interface and provides more secure fixation.[5,28,29] An important technical consideration when performing single-row repairs is to use mattress, Mason-Allen, massive cuff stitch, or comparable suture configurations to improve the biomechanical strength of the repair (**Fig. 2**). In 2 separate biomechanical studies, Lorbach and colleagues[28,29] reported single-row repairs using a modified mattress suture configuration with either double-loaded or triple-loaded anchors were similar in load to failure and cyclic displacement to a double-row suture-bridge technique independent of the tested tear sizes; however, the double-row repair consistently restored a larger footprint than the single-row configurations. Additional studies have reported similar outcomes for cyclic failure and footprint restoration using modified Mason-Allen or massive cuff stitch single-row suture anchor techniques. Simple suture configurations with single-row repairs have demonstrated inferior biomechanical properties and footprint coverage in all of these studies.[30,31]

Single-row repairs have been shown to inadequately restore tendon coverage over the RTC footprint when compared with double-row and transosseous-equivalent techniques. Meier and Meier[32] reported double-row suture anchor fixation

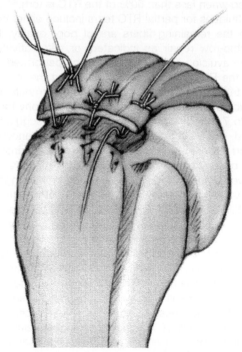

Fig. 2. Diagram illustrating the arthroscopic modified Mason-Allen technique for RTC repair using a single row of suture anchors. (*Data from* Scheibel MT, Habermeyer P. A modified Mason-Allen technique for RTC repair using suture anchors. Arthroscopy 2003;19(3):330–3; with permission.)

consistently restored 100% of the native supraspinatus footprint, whereas the single-row suture anchor fixation restored 46%. In a clinical study of 26 patients undergoing arthroscopic RTC repair, Brady and colleagues[33] reported isolated single-row repairs left 52.7% of the RTC footprint uncovered.

Although individual studies may report better clinical outcomes with double-row repair constructs, collectively, the literature has not definitively proved superior results with regard to pain relief or functional outcomes, particularly in tears less than 3 cm in size.[17,34–38] A systematic review by Duquin and colleagues[39] concluded that double-row repair methods lead to significantly lower retear rates compared with single-row methods for tears greater than 1 cm. A clinical study by Charousset and colleagues[40] of 66 patients undergoing arthroscopic RTC repair with either single-row or double-row techniques found no significant difference in clinical results, but tendon healing rates were better with the double-row technique.

Logistical considerations for use of single-row techniques over double-row or transosseous-equivalent techniques are increased cost, longer surgical time, and increased technical demand of these newer methods.[9,10,29,34,35] Single-row repairs, using double-loaded or triple-loaded anchors with modified mattress configurations, may provide predictable success of clinical outcomes in patients with small to medium RTC tears.[9,10,34,39]

Double-Row and Transosseous Equivalent

Double-row suture anchor repair techniques involve placing a medial row of anchors at the humeral head articular margin and a second row of anchors laterally on the footprint (**Fig. 3**). Each suture anchor provides an independent point of fixation. Lo and

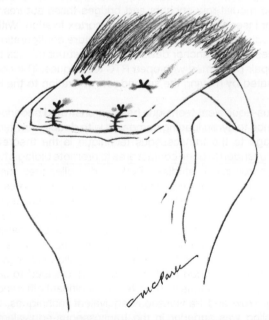

Fig. 3. Diagram illustrating a double-row suture anchor technique with medial row anchors placed in a horizontal mattress configuration and the lateral row of anchors with simple sutures. (*From* Park MC, Pirolo JM, Park CJ, et al. The effect of abduction and rotation on footprint contact for single-row, double-row, and modified double-row rotator cuff repair techniques. Am J Sports Med 2009;37(8):1599–608; with permission.)

Burkhart[20] described the technique using horizontal mattress sutures tied medially and simple sutures tied laterally. It is important to assure the tendon is of adequate size and mobility when using this construct to prevent excessive strain on the repair site.

As discussed previously, double-row repairs routinely restore coverage of the RTC footprint to a greater extent than single-row constructs.[32,33,41] The increased footprint coverage of double-row repairs theoretically provides a greater surface area for tendon to bone healing to occur. Biomechanical studies consistently report decreased gap formation, increased cyclic load to failure, and increased ultimate load to failure.[31,42–44]

In a systematic review, DeHaan and colleagues[17] reported retear rate of 43.1% for the single-row repair and 27.2% for the double-row repair although this difference was not statistically significant. Another systematic review by Saradakis and Jones[34] concluded double-row repairs result in improved structural healing but no significant clinical differences in clinical outcomes when compared with single-row constructs in less than 3-cm RTC tears. A third systematic review by Duquin and colleagues[39] concluded double-row repair methods lead to significantly lower retear rates when compared with single-row methods for tears greater than 1 cm. A recent prospective, randomized trial of 53 patients by Ma and colleagues[45] found arthroscopic RTC repair with double-row fixation resulted in better shoulder strength in patients with greater than 3 cm tears compared with single-row methods, although there was no significant difference in RTC integrity in either groups in patients with any tear size at a minimum 2-year follow-up.

Disadvantages of the double-row technique include increased cost, operating room time, increased technical difficulty, potential for anchor crowding within the footprint, synovial fluid leakage at the repair site, and point fixation at the repair site versus a broad surface area contact.[9,10,46–48] Because of these concerns, Park and colleagues[9] developed a transosseous-equivalent RTC repair that preserves the suture limbs of the medial row anchors and bridges these sutures over the greater tuberosity footprint insertion with lateral humeral cortex fixation. With this technique, the medial row of sutures is passed in a mattress suture configuration that is secured laterally with knotless suture anchor devices. The construct mimics the classic transosseous suture repair performed with open RTC techniques. The concern for anchor crowding is eliminated by moving the second row of fixation to the lateral wall of the tuberosity.

The transosseous-equivalent technique has demonstrated superior ultimate load to failure and resistance to cyclic loading compared with double-row techniques.[46,47] An additional advantage to the transosseous technique is the theoretic advantage of providing increased tendon to bone contact area to promote biologic healing. In a series of cadaveric biomechanical studies, Park and colleagues demonstrated the transosseous-equivalent repair technique had the highest pressurized footprint coverage and stronger mean load to failure in biomechanical testing at time zero when compared with double-row techniques. The transosseous technique showed 77.6% of the anatomic footprint had pressurized coverage compared with 39.6% for the double-row construct. Mazzocca and colleagues[49] reported the contact pressure at the footprint was highest at all time points with cyclic loading with the transosseous-equivalent repairs, although contact pressure decreased to some extent in all constructs. Behrens and colleagues[50] reported no significant differences in gap formation between single-row and transosseous-equivalent techniques, although fixation strength after cycling was superior in the transosseous-equivalent configurations. The majority of gapping occurred in all constructs during the first 100 cycles.

Synovial fluid leakage into the tendon-bone interface of an RTC repair may potentially impede healing. Compared with a double-row repair, the transosseous-equivalent water-tight technique was shown by Nassos and colleagues[48] to significantly decrease the leakage of synovial fluid into the footprint of the RTC repair construct using a cadaveric external rotation model and a pressurized gelatin technique. Only one study has formally assessed the tendon vascularity of the transosseous-equivalent technique. In a clinical study of 18 patients, Christoforetti and colleagues[51] performed recordings with a custom laser Doppler flowmetry probe to determine the overall effect on blood flow associated with this technique. The investigators demonstrated a significant (44.67%) decline in the blood flow present after the second row of implants was placed. The clinical implications of this reduced, but preserved, blood flow are yet to be determined.

There are several key technical pearls when using the transosseous-equivalent technique for RTC repair. First is to ensure the tendon has been appropriately mobilized so the tendon is not overtensioned at the repair site. There should be easy excursion of the tendon over the tuberosity. Second, it should be confirmed that there is sufficient tendon to place 2 rows of anchors to appropriately plan for suture placement. Park and colleagues[9] recommend inserting the lateral fixation points 1 cm distal-lateral to the lateral edge of the tuberosity footprint insertion.

Recent studies have stressed the importance of tying knots at the medial row of mattress sutures before tensioning laterally (**Fig. 4**).[52–55] Variations of transosseous-equivalent constructs have been marketed that propose a technically easier and faster surgery by eliminating the need for any knot tying. This technique passes the medial row of sutures but does not require tying any knots at the medial row. Investigators have hypothesized that tying medial row knots is important to protect the supraspinatus footprint area by resisting gap formation, increasing the yield load, ultimate load, and the energy absorbed by the construct in failure loading.[52,55]

In a controlled laboratory study, Busfield and colleagues[52] randomized 6 matched pairs of cadaveric shoulders into 2 groups of transosseous-equvialent fixation with

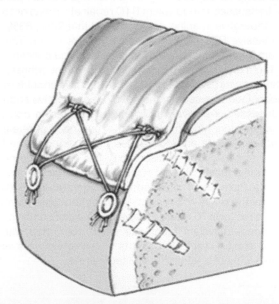

Fig. 4. Diagram depicting a transosseous-equivalent RTC repair. The image demonstrates the technique of tying knots at the medial row horizontal mattress sutures. (*From* Pauly S, Kieser B, Schill A, et al. Biomechanical comparison of 4 double-row suture-bridging rotator cuff repair techniques using different medial-row configurations. Arthroscopy 2010;26(10):1281–8; with permission.)

a suture-bridge technique. One group was fixed with medial row knots and another without medial row knots. The medial row knot group had statistically significant results for preventing gap formation at all cyclic load time points. In addition, there was greater energy absorbed (2805 vs 1648 N-mm), yield load (233 vs 183.1 N), and ultimate load (352.9 N vs 253.9 N) for the medial row knot group. In a porcine shoulder model, Pauly and colleagues[54] concluded application of a suture-bridge repair with double medial mattress stitches significantly enhanced biomechanical initial stability and resistance to suture cutting through the RTC. In a cadaveric shoulder external rotation model, Kaplan and colleagues[55] also found adding an additional horizontal mattress suture with medial knots separate sutures in the medial-row anchors helps to neutralize forces experienced by the repair. Modifications of the transosseous-equivalent technique, such as the diamondback configuration, have been further devised to enhance the pressurized contact area of the tendon to bone.[56]

When introducing a new technique, it is important to consider the complications or modes of failure that present themselves after clinical use. Dierckman and colleagues[53] studied the maximum load and point of failure of the construct during tensioning of the lateral row of a transosseous-equivalent RTC. The study concluded caution is necessary when tensioning the lateral row as failure occurred most commonly at the polyetheretherketone eyelets of knotless anchor implants. Other studies have shown the primary site of failure with double-row and transosseous-equivalent repair is at the musculotendinous junction.[10,54,55,57] When failure occurs at this location, it presents a complex revision scenario. This should be considered before using the transosseous-equivalent technique. Preventative strategies include avoidance of overtensioning the medial row and placing the medial row of sutures lateral to the musculotendinous junction near the RTC cable.[10]

Initial clinical studies have shown promising results for the transosseous-equivalent technique. Toussaint and colleagues[58] reported the results of 154 patients who underwent arthroscopic transosseous-equivalent RTC repair at a mean of 15 months' follow-up. Analysis of postoperative imaging demonstrated that 92%, 83%, and 84% of the small, large, and massive RTC tears, respectively, were intact. The mean Constant score improved from 44.42 points to 80.47 points. Kim and colleagues[59] reported 52 consecutive RTC 1 mm to 4 cm in dimension that underwent arthroscopic RTC repair. A double-row technique was used in the first 26 consecutive shoulders, and a transosseous-equivalent technique was used in the next 26 consecutive shoulders. The study concluded the transosseous-equivalent technique resulted in comparable, but not superior, patient satisfaction, functional outcome, and rates of retear compared with double-row techniques. Mihata and colleagues[60] has reported the largest series of patients with the longest follow-up to date. Sixty-five RTCs were repaired using the single-row, 23 using the double-row, and 107 using the transosseous-equivalent techniques with an average follow up of 38.5 months. Retear rates were 10.8%, 26.1%, and 4.7%, respectively, for the single-row, double-row, and transosseous-equivalent techniques. The large and massive RTC tear groups had a significantly lower rate of retear using the transosseous-equivalent technique when compared with the single-row group. Postoperative clinical results in patients with a retear were significantly lower than those in patients without a retear for all 3 techniques.

SUMMARY

Techniques for arthroscopic partial-thickness and full-thickness RTC repairs continue to advance. When selecting an RTC repair technique, it is important to identify the tear pattern and adhere to the fundamentals of tendon mobilization and footprint preparation.

Partial RTC tears greater than 50% in thickness can be reproducibly repaired with tear completion or transtendinous techniques with good clinical outcomes. Based on the available literature, small, less than 1-cm RTC tears can effectively be repaired with single-row techniques. Tears sized 1 cm to 3 cm can be repaired with either single-row, double-row, or transosseous-equivalent techniques based on surgeon comfort, tendon quality, and tissue mobility. Tears greater than 3 cm have shown superior results when transosseous-equivalent techniques are used. Further clinical studies are needed to definitively conclude the ideal RTC repair technique.

REFERENCES

1. Abrams JS, Savoie FH III. Arthroscopic rotator cuff repair: is it the new gold standard? 72nd Annual Meeting Proceedings. Rosemont (IL): American Academy of Orthopaedic Surgeons; 2005. p. 71.
2. Dunn WR, Schackman BR, Walsh C, et al. Variation in orthopaedic surgeons' perceptions about the indications for rotator cuff surgery. J Bone Joint Surg Am 2005;87(9):1978–84.
3. Colvin AC, Egorova N, Harrison AK, et al. National trends in rotator cuff repair. J Bone Joint Surg Am 2012;94(3):227–33.
4. Ellman H. Diagnosis and treatment of incomplete rotator cuff tears. Clin Orthop Relat Res 1990;254:64–74.
5. Burkhart SS, Lo IK. Arthroscopic rotator cuff repair. J Am Acad Orthop Surg 2006; 14(6):333–46.
6. Dugas JR, Campbell DA, Warren RF, et al. Anatomy and dimensions of rotator cuff insertions. J Shoulder Elbow Surg 2002;11(5):498–503.
7. Mochizuki T, Sugaya H, Uomizu M, et al. Humeral insertion of the supraspinatus and infraspinatus. New anatomical findings regarding the footprint of the rotator cuff. J Bone Joint Surg Am 2008;90(5):962–9.
8. Goutallier D, Postel JM, Bernageau J, et al. Fatty muscle degeneration in cuff ruptures. Pre- and postoperative evaluation by CT scan. Clin Orthop Relat Res 1994;304:78–83.
9. Park MC, Elattrache NS, Ahmad CS, et al. "Transosseous-equivalent" rotator cuff repair technique. Arthroscopy 2006;22(12):1360.e1–5.
10. Provencher MT, Kercher JS, Galatz LM, et al. Evolution of rotator cuff repair techniques: are our patients really benefiting? Instr Course Lect 2011;60:123–36.
11. Levy O, Venkateswaran B, Even T, et al. Midterm clinical and sonographic outcome of arthroscopic repair of the rotator cuff. J Bone Joint Surg Am 2008;90:1341–7.
12. Bishop J, Klepps S, Lo IK, et al. Cuff integrity after arthroscopic versus open rotator cuff repair: a prospective study. J Shoulder Elbow Surg 2006;15(3):290–9.
13. Galatz LM, Ball CM, Teefey SA, et al. The outcome and repair integrity of completely arthroscopically repaired large and massive rotator cuff tears. J Bone Joint Surg Am 2004;86:219–24.
14. Boileau P, Brassart N, Watkinson DJ, et al. Arthroscopic repair of full-thickness tears of the supraspinatus: does the tendon really heal? J Bone Joint Surg Am 2005;87(6):1229–40.
15. Cole BJ, McCarty LP 3rd, Kang RW, et al. Arthroscopic rotator cuff repair: prospective functional outcome and repair integrity at minimum 2-year follow-up. J Shoulder Elbow Surg 2007;16(5):579–85.
16. Sugaya H, Maeda K, Matsuki K, et al. Repair integrity and functional outcome after arthroscopic double-row rotator cuff repair. A prospective outcome study. J Bone Joint Surg Am 2007;89(5):953–60.

17. DeHaan AM, Axelrad TW, Kaye E, et al. Does double-row rotator cuff repair improve functional outcome of patients compared with single-row technique? A systematic review. Am J Sports Med 2012;40(5):1176–85.
18. Slabaugh MA, Nho SJ, Grumet RC, et al. Does the literature confirm superior clinical results in radiographically healed rotator cuffs after rotator cuff repair? Arthroscopy 2010;26(3):393–403.
19. Jost B, Pfirrmann CW, Gerber C. Clinical outcome after structural failure of rotator cuff repairs. J Bone Joint Surg Am 2000;82:304–14.
20. Lo IK, Burkhart SS. Double-row arthroscopic rotator cuff repair: re-establishing the footprint of the rotator cuff. Arthroscopy 2003;19(9):1035–42.
21. Mazzocca AD, Rincon LM, O'Connor RW, et al. Intra-articular partial-thickness rotator cuff tears: analysis of injured and repaired strain behavior. Am J Sports Med 2008;36(1):110–6.
22. Yamanaka K, Matsumoto T. The joint side tear of the rotator cuff. A followup study by arthrography. Clin Orthop Relat Res 1994;304:68–73.
23. Duralde XA, McClelland WB Jr. The clinical results of arthroscopic transtendinous repair of grade III partial articular-sided supraspinatus tendon tears. Arthroscopy 2012;28(2):160–8.
24. Franceschi F, Papalia R, Del Buono A, et al. Repair of partial tears of the rotator cuff. Sports Med Arthrosc 2011;19(4):401–8.
25. Shin SJ. A comparison of 2 repair techniques for partial-thickness articular-sided rotator cuff tears. Arthroscopy 2012;28(1):25–33.
26. Strauss EJ, Salata MJ, Kercher J, et al. Multimedia article. The arthroscopic management of partial-thickness rotator cuff tears: a systematic review of the literature. Arthroscopy 2011;27(4):568–80 Review.
27. Kibler WB, Sciascia A, Wolf BR, et al. Nonacute shoulder injuries. In: Kibler W, editor. Orthopaedic knowledge update 4. Sports medicine. Rosemont, IL: American Academy of Orthopaedic Surgeons; 2009. p. 19–39.
28. Lorbach O, Bachelier F, Vees J, et al. Cyclic loading of rotator cuff reconstructions: single-row repair with modified suture configurations versus double-row repair. Am J Sports Med 2008;36(8):1504–10.
29. Lorbach O, Kieb M, Raber F, et al. Comparable biomechanical results for a modified single-row rotator cuff reconstruction using triple-loaded suture anchors versus a suture-bridging double-row repair. Arthroscopy 2012;28(2):178–87.
30. Ma CB, Comerford L, Wilson J, et al. Biomechanical evaluation of arthroscopic rotator cuff repairs: double-row compared with single-row fixation. J Bone Joint Surg Am 2006;88:403–10.
31. Baums MH, Spahn G, Steckel H, et al. Comparative evaluation of the tendon-bone interface contact pressure in different single- versus double-row suture anchor repair techniques. Knee Surg Sports Traumatol Arthrosc 2009;17: 1466–72.
32. Meier SW, Meier JD. Rotator cuff repair: the effect of double-row fixation on three-dimensional repair site. J Shoulder Elbow Surg 2006;15(6):691–6.
33. Brady PC, Arrigoni P, Burkhart SS. Evaluation of residual rotator cuff defects after in vivo single- versus double-row rotator cuff repairs. Arthroscopy 2006;22(10): 1070–5.
34. Saridakis P, Jones G. Outcomes of single-row and double-row arthroscopic rotator cuff repair: a systematic review. J Bone Joint Surg Am 2010;92(3):732–42 Review.
35. Franceschi F, Ruzzini L, Longo UG, et al. Equivalent clinical results of arthroscopic single-row and double-row suture anchor repair for rotator cuff tears: a randomized controlled trial. Am J Sports Med 2007;35:1254–60.

36. Burks RT, Crim J, Brown N, et al. A prospective randomized clinical trial comparing arthroscopic single- and double-row rotator cuff repair: magnetic resonance imaging and early clinical evaluation. Am J Sports Med 2009;37:674–82.
37. Aydin N, Kocaoglu B, Guven O. Single-row versus double row arthroscopic rotator cuff repair in small- to medium-sized tears. J Shoulder Elbow Surg 2010;19:722–5.
38. Koh KH, Kang KC, Lim TK, et al. Prospective randomized clinical trial of single-versus double-row suture anchor repair in 2- to 4-cm rotator cuff tears: clinical and magnetic resonance imaging results. Arthroscopy 2011;27:453–62.
39. Duquin TR, Buyea C, Bisson LJ. Which method of rotator cuff repair leads to the highest rate of structural healing? A systematic review. Am J Sports Med 2010; 38(4):835–41 Review.
40. Charousset C, Grimberg J, Duranthon LD, et al. Can a double-row anchorage technique improve tendon healing in arthroscopic rotator cuff repair? A prospective, nonrandomized, comparative study of double-row and single-row anchorage techniques with computed tomographic arthrography tendon healing assessment. Am J Sports Med 2007;35:1247–53.
41. Mazzocca AD, Millet PJ, Guanche CA, et al. Arthroscopic single-row versus double-row suture anchor rotator cuff repair. Am J Sports Med 2005;33:1861–8.
42. Kim DH, ElAttrache NS, Tibone JE, et al. Biomechanical comparison of a single-row versus double-row suture anchor technique for rotator cuff repair. Am J Sports Med 2006;34:407–14.
43. Milano G, Grasso A, Zarelli D, et al. Comparison between single-row and double-row rotator cuff repair: a biomechanical study. Knee Surg Sports Traumatol Arthrosc 2008;16:75–80.
44. Smith CD, Alexander S, Hill AM, et al. A biomechanical comparison of single and double-row fixation in arthroscopic rotator cuff repair. J Bone Joint Surg Am 2006; 88:2425–31.
45. Ma HL, Chiang ER, Wu HT, et al. Clinical outcome and imaging of arthroscopic single-row and double-row rotator cuff repair: a prospective randomized trial. Arthroscopy 2012;28(1):16–24.
46. Park MC, Tibone JE, ElAttrache NS, et al. Part II: biomechanical assessment for a footprint-restoring transosseous-equivalent rotator cuff repair technique compared with a double-row repair technique. J Shoulder Elbow Surg 2007; 16(4):469–76.
47. Park MC, ElAttrache NS, Tibone JE, et al. Part I: footprint contact characteristics for a transosseous-equivalent rotator cuff repair technique compared with a double-row repair technique. J Shoulder Elbow Surg 2007;16(4):461–8.
48. Nassos JT, Elattrache NS, Angel MJ, et al. A watertight construct in arthroscopic rotator cuff repair. J Shoulder Elbow Surg 2012;21(5):589–96.
49. Mazzocca AD, Bollier MJ, Ciminiello AM, et al. Biomechanical evaluation of arthroscopic rotator cuff repairs over time. Arthroscopy 2010;26:592–9.
50. Behrens SB, Bruce B, Zonno AJ, et al. Initial fixation strength of transosseous-equivalent suture bridge rotator cuff repair is comparable with transosseous repair. Am J Sports Med 2012;40(1):133–40.
51. Christoforetti JJ, Krupp RJ, Singleton SB, et al. Arthroscopic suture bridge transosseous equivalent fixation of rotator cuff tendon preserves intratendinous blood flow at the time of initial fixation. J Shoulder Elbow Surg 2012;21(4):523–30.
52. Busfield BT, Glousman RE, McGarry MH, et al. A biomechanical comparison of 2 technical variations of double-row rotator cuff fixation: the importance of medial row knots. Am J Sports Med 2008;36(5):901–6.

53. Dierckman BD, Goldstein JL, Hammond KE, et al. A biomechanical analysis of point of failure during lateral-row tensioning in transosseous-equivalent rotator cuff repair. Arthroscopy 2012;28(1):52–8.
54. Pauly S, Kieser B, Schill A, et al. Biomechanical comparison of 4 double-row suture-bridging rotator cuff repair techniques using different medial-row configurations. Arthroscopy 2010;26(10):1281–8.
55. Kaplan K, ElAttrache NS, Vazquez O, et al. Knotless rotator cuff repair in an external rotation model: the importance of medial-row horizontal mattress sutures. Arthroscopy 2011;27(4):471–8.
56. Burkhart SS, Denard PJ, Obopilwe E, et al. Optimizing pressurized contact area in rotator cuff repair: the diamondback repair. Arthroscopy 2012;28(2):188–95.
57. Cho NS, Yi JW, Lee BG, et al. Retear patterns after arthroscopic rotator cuff repair: single-row versus suture bridge technique. Am J Sports Med 2010;38(4):664–71.
58. Toussaint B, Schnaser E, Bosley J, et al. Early structural and functional outcomes for arthroscopic double-row transosseous-equivalent rotator cuff repair. Am J Sports Med 2011;39(6):1217–25.
59. Kim KC, Shin HD, Lee WY, et al. Repair integrity and functional outcome after arthroscopic rotator cuff repair: double-row versus suture-bridge technique. Am J Sports Med 2012;40(2):294–9.
60. Mihata T, Watanabe C, Fukunishi K, et al. Functional and structural outcomes of single-row versus double-row versus combined double-row and suture-bridge repair for rotator cuff tears. Am J Sports Med 2011;39(10):2091–8.

Biologics in the Management of Rotator Cuff Surgery

Michael E. Angeline, MD[a,b], Scott A. Rodeo, MD[a,b],*

KEYWORDS

- Tendon biology • Bone morphogenetic protein • Growth factors • Repair scaffolds

KEY POINTS

- Surgical repair of rotator cuff tears is a relatively common orthopedic procedure.
- Although the procedure is clinically successful, the repair site frequently has incomplete healing and gap formation, owing to a fibrovascular scar–mediated healing response at the tendon-bone interface.
- By augmenting the repair site with biological agents, the ultimate goal is to stimulate a regenerative healing pathway.

INTRODUCTION

Rotator cuff tears constitute a widespread problem that causes significant pain and disability. Arthroscopic surgical repair has thus become increasingly common. The results of arthroscopic full-thickness repair have been shown to be comparable with those obtained with open or mini-open techniques.[1] Despite clinical success rates of more than 85% after rotator cuff repair, persistent anatomic defects remain, with incomplete healing and gap formation, which is likely related to the size of the tear repaired and age of the patient.[2–4] In addition, it has been shown that functional results after repair are superior in patients with intact rotator cuffs at follow-up.[5,6] Consequently there has been much interest in developing novel treatments to improve the healing rates and functional outcomes after rotator cuff repairs, because the healing process results in a reactive scar rather than a histologically normal tendon-bone insertion site.

Many studies have investigated methods to strengthen rotator cuff repairs by using stronger sutures and restoring the anatomic footprint. These methods are still associated with substantial failure rates, with retears occurring in up to 50% of patients.[7]

The authors have nothing to disclose.
^a Department of Orthopaedic Surgery, Hospital for Special Surgery, New York, NY, USA;
^b Sports Medicine and Shoulder Surgery Service, Hospital for Special Surgery, 535 East 70th Street, New York, NY 10021, USA
* Corresponding author.
E-mail address: rodeos@hss.edu

Clin Sports Med 31 (2012) 645–663
http://dx.doi.org/10.1016/j.csm.2012.07.003
0278-5919/12/$ – see front matter © 2012 Elsevier Inc. All rights reserved.

More recently studies have focused on biological augmentation of rotator cuff repairs.[2,8–10] In this review the use of biologics to improve healing of the tendon-bone insertion site after a repair is evaluated. First, however, the developmental biology of the rotator cuff enthesis and the histology/biology that occurs during the healing process is examined. It is important to keep in mind that the structure formed after a repair does not reestablish the native tendon insertion site that was formed during embryologic development.

The normal tendon-bone insertion site is composed of 4 distinct transition zones: tendon, fibrocartilage, mineralized fibrocartilage, and bone.[11] The fundamental function of the insertion site is to minimize stress concentration at the junction between soft tissue (tendon) and hard tissue (bone). The collagen content of these transition zones differs based on the tissue type. The tendinous portion is primarily composed of type I and III collagen while the fibrocartilaginous zone is composed of types I, II, and III collagen. The mineralized fibrocartilage zone contains types I, II, and X collagen. The final bone portion of the enthesis consists of type I collagen (**Fig. 1**).[12,13]

Tendon healing does not regenerate the tendon-bone interface that was formed during prenatal development. Instead, healing results in a fibrovascular scar at the interface that is mechanically weaker than the native insertion site and more prone to failure.[14,15] This scarring occurs through a 3-phase process of inflammation, repair, and remodeling (**Fig. 2**).[11,14]

Within the early stages of the inflammatory phase, fibrin and fibronectin are initially deposited by platelets. Macrophages then accumulate in response to cytokine-mediated signaling from insulin-like growth factor 1 (IGF-1), platelet- derived growth factor (PDGF), and transforming growth factor β (TGF-β). The macrophages then secrete TGF-β1, which marks the transition into the repair phase resulting in fibroblastic proliferation and formation of scar tissue.

The newly formed scar tissue, which is composed of primarily type III collagen, then undergoes matrix metalloproteinase (MMP)-mediated remodeling as a result of extracellular mediated turnover.[16]

In contrast to the postnatal healing response, fetal wound healing occurs through a "scarless" process. It is theorized that this is due to absence of an inflammatory response, an absence of mechanical load on the healing tendon, and a large number of undifferentiated cells at the healing interface. Given this absence of an inflammatory response, there are molecular signals and cellular differentiation events not present within the postnatal organism.[17] Galatz and colleagues[12] found that TGF-β1

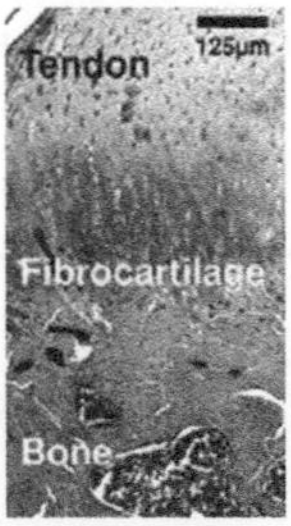

Tissue Region	Cell Type	Major Matrix Component
Tendon	Fibroblasts	Collagen types I, III (Diameter: 40-400 nm)*
Non-mineralized Fibrocartilage	Fibrochondrocytes	Collagen types I, II, III
Mineralized Fibrocartilage	Hypertrophic Fibrochondrocytes	Collagen types I, II, X
Bone	Osteoblasts Osteocytes Osteoclasts	Collagen type I (Diameter: 34.5-39.5nm)^

Fig. 1. The structure and composition of the 4 zones comprising the direct tendon-to-bone insertion site. (*From* Zhang X, Bogdanowicz D, Eriksen C, et al. Biomimetic scaffold design for functional and integrative tendon repair. J Shoulder Elbow Surg 2012;21(2):266–77; with permission.)

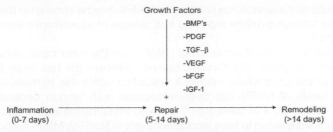

Growth Factors
-BMP's
-PDGF
-TGF-β
-VEGF
-bFGF
-IGF-1
+

Inflammation ————————→ Repair ————————→ Remodeling
(0-7 days)   (5-14 days)   (>14 days)

Fig. 2. The stages of rotator cuff healing involve inflammation, repair, and remodeling. Growth factors are expressed during the repair phase, because they promote cell proliferation and matrix production. This timeline must be kept in mind in growth-factor therapies, because the addition of growth factors too early or late in the healing process may decrease their effectiveness. bFGF, basic fibroblast growth factor; BMP, bone morphogenetic protein; IGF-1, insulin-like growth factor 1; PDGF, platelet-derived growth factor; TGF-β, transforming growth factor β; VEGF, vascular endothelial growth factor. (*Reprinted from* Gulotta LV, Rodeo SA. Growth factors for rotator cuff repair. Clin Sports Med 2009;28(1):13–23.)

expression was turned on and TGF-β3 was turned off 15.5 days after conception within the developing supraspinatus tendon in a murine model. This time point coincides with the end of the regenerative healing pathway and the beginning of the scar-mediated pathway.

To explore this further, Kobayashi and colleagues[18] and Würgler-Hauri and colleagues[19] examined the expression of growth factors during the healing of acute rotator cuff tears. Kobayashi and colleagues noted that there was a sequential expression of basic fibroblast growth factor (bFGF), IGF-1, PDGF, and TGF-β within acutely injured supraspinatus tendons of Japanese white rabbits. Würgler-Hauri and colleagues also noted a temporal expression of bFGF, bone morphogenetic protein (BMP)-12, BMP-13, BMP-14, cartilage oligomeric matrix protein (COMP), connective tissue growth factor (CTGF), PDGF, and TGF-β1. From these studies in animal models it can be seen that the cytokines involved in tendon healing play major and overall positive roles in cell proliferation, chemotaxis, differentiation, and matrix synthesis.

Using the gene-expression patterns of these cytokines, the ultimate goal is to recreate the native tendon insertion site, which was formed during embryologic development, and improve rotator cuff tendon healing. The main challenges that exist, however, are identification of the optimal factors, the ideal timing of delivery, and the ideal delivery vehicle.

The purpose of this review is to examine the current state of biological agents and their use for augmentation of rotator cuff tendon healing. The reader should be able to gain an understanding of the various growth factors, supplements, and tissue-engineering techniques that could be potentially useful in improving the biology of rotator cuff healing.

THE ROLE OF MATRIX METALLOPROTEINASES AND THEIR INHIBITORS IN TENDON-BONE HEALING

Recent studies have shown that matrix metalloproteinases (MMPs) and their inhibitors may play a critical role in the pathophysiology of rotator cuff tears.[20] The MMPs, specifically MMP-1, MMP-8, and MMP-13, are a family of at least 24 zinc-dependent endopeptidases that are responsible for the degradation of the extracellular matrix including the fibrillar collagens, which provide mechanical strength to tissues.[20] Additional research has shown that MMPs may be involved in the inflammatory response through cytokine signaling and release of neoepitopes from the extracellular matrix.[21]

Tissue inhibitors of metalloproteinases (TIMPs), on the other hand, antagonize the effects of MMP enzymes. The dynamic balance between the two helps to maintain the integrity of the extracellular matrix. A disruption within this homeostasis leading to elevated levels of MMPs has been associated with tendon degeneration and rupture.[22,23] Pasternak and colleagues[24] showed that patients with an acute Achilles tendon rupture were noted to have increased levels of MMP-2, MMP-7, and TIMP-2 in the serum.

Looking specifically at full-thickness rotator cuff tears, Lo and colleagues[25] found elevated mRNA levels of the collagenase MMP-13 and decreased mRNA levels of the stromelysin MMP-3 as well as TIMP-2, TIMP-3, and TIMP-4. Yoshihara also noted elevated levels of MMP-1, MMP-3, and glycosaminoglycans within the synovial fluid of patients with massive rotator cuff tears.[26] Further work by McDowell and colleagues[27] has shown that MMP-mediated tissue degradation within the immediate postoperative period after a surgical repair leads to weakening of the tendon around the suture construct.

Based on the involvement of MMP-TIMP systems in tendon degeneration, recent research has explored the possibility that selective inhibition of MMPs may have a positive effect on tendon healing.[20] Several pharmacologic classes of MMP inhibitors exist; however, doxycycline is considered to be the most potent MMP inhibitor. Its nonantibiotic mechanism of action includes binding to the zinc-binding site of the MMP enzyme and inhibition of MMP gene expression, specifically inhibiting MMPs 1, 2, 7, 8, 9, 12, and 13.[20]

With this concept in mind, Pasternak and colleagues[28] demonstrated in a rat Achilles tendon model that doxycycline-coated sutures improved holding capacity for early tendon suture. Further work from the authors' laboratory has shown that doxycycline-mediated inhibition of MMP-13 activity after an acute rotator cuff repair was associated with improvements in both biomechanical and histologic parameters of healing at the tendon-bone interface in a rat model.[22] Although further research needs to be done to determine the exact mechanism by which MMP inhibition leads to improved tendon-to-bone healing, this treatment modality may become a therapeutic alternative for augmentation of rotator cuff repairs.

ANGIOGENESIS AND ANGIOGENIC CYTOKINES IN ROTATOR CUFF REPAIRS

Work by Brooks and colleagues[29] identified the distal 15 mm of the supraspinatus and infraspinatus tendons adjacent to the distal insertion site as a relative hypovascular area. The investigators implicated this area as a potential source of tendon degeneration; therefore, a logical tenet of tendon repair is to reestablish the vascularity at the tendon-bone interface. However, there still remains a paucity of data to support or refute the claim that a failure to reestablish this vascularity leads to poor tendon healing. Based on this concept, work by others at the authors' institution has examined the vascularity of the supraspinatus tendon after repair using power Doppler sonography.[30–32]

The first in this series of studies prospectively examined rotator cuff repairs at 6 weeks, 3 months, and 6 months postoperatively using power Doppler sonography.[31]

Several repair techniques were used within this cohort, but despite this confounding factor the findings of the study consistently showed that there was an initial robust vascular response after repair, which diminished with time. The peritendinous region showed the highest vascular response at each time point while the site of the bony bed to which the tendon was repaired had the lowest vascular scores. Of interest, it was also demonstrated that the vascular scores of the repaired tendons were similar whether or not a defect was noted on ultrasonography postoperatively. In addition, the vascular scores were consistently low in all regions of the rotator cuff within asymptomatic control patients. These findings suggest that the vascularity and biology of the tendon repair is unclear.

In 2 subsequent follow-up studies, contrast-enhanced ultrasonography was used to examine the vascularity of the supraspinatus tendon 3 months and at a minimum of 10 months after repair.[30,32] At the 3-month time point after repair, the supraspinatus tendon itself was found to be relatively avascular, with the surrounding peribursal soft tissues and anchor site serving as the main sources of blood flow to the repair site.[32] The same patient cohort showed similar vascular patterns at longer postoperative follow-up, in addition to exercise-enhanced vascular perfusion to the peribursal area.[30] These findings suggest that the tendon's surrounding vascular environment may potentially influence healing of the repair site.[32]

With the characterization of the vascular response at the tendon repair site in mind, there has been renewed interest recently in research into proinflammatory/angiogenic cytokines. Cytokines influence cell proliferation, differentiation, and matrix synthesis during the tendon-healing process. Although no specific study has clearly shown that improved vascularity will result in improved tendon healing, an understanding and use of the growth factors involved in the healing response may potentially lead to improved healing. The great difficulty that still exists, however, is to identify the dosing, timing, and delivery methods for the growth factors either in isolation or in combination.

Vascular endothelial growth factor (VEGF) is a general term that covers a family of signaling proteins including placenta growth factor and VEGF-A, -B, -C, and -D.[33] The most important factor within this family is VEGF-A, but all function to stimulate both angiogenesis and vasculogenesis through a tyrosine kinase receptor–mediated signaling cascade. No specific study has been done examining VEGF augmentation of rotator cuff repairs, although work has been done examining the effects of VEGF on flexor and Achilles tendon healing models as well as sheep anterior cruciate ligament (ACL) reconstruction models.[34–36]

Using in situ hybridization techniques, Bidder and colleagues[34] examined the location of cell populations that contribute to the neovascularization process through expression of VEGF in a canine flexor tendon repair model. This study showed that the majority of cells at and around the tenorrhaphy site expressed VEGF, and therefore contributed to the organization of the angiogenic response during the early postoperative phase of tendon healing. In a rat Achilles tendon model, exogenous VEGF was injected into the repair site, and during the early postoperative period (1 and 2 weeks) there was increased tensile strength in the VEGF treatment group compared with controls.[35] This finding further supports the potential benefit of VEGF augmentation in the early stages of tendon healing.

In contrast to these results, application of VEGF in a sheep ACL reconstruction model showed lower stiffness and increased laxity of the femur-graft-tibia complex in comparison with the control group.[36] Histologic findings showed increased angiogenesis and vascularity in the VEGF-soaked treatment group compared with control grafts soaked in phosphate-buffered saline. Although these results show a potentially negative effect of VEGF on ACL graft healing, only one time point was evaluated within this study (12 weeks postoperative), and it is unclear whether these findings can be extrapolated to rotator cuff healing.

In addition to VEGF, fibroblast growth factors (FGFs) also act as angiogenic cytokines whose application could be used to promote tendon healing in a rotator cuff repair. The FGFs are a family of 23 structurally related polypeptides that have an affinity to heparin-binding sites on target cells.[37] Their main function is to stimulate angiogenesis through proliferation of capillary endothelial cells, and they also have a mitogenic effect on mesenchymal cells.[11,33] In adult tissue, FGF-1 (or acidic FGF) and FGF-2 (basic FGF) are the most abundant. While both are present early within the repair process, FGF-2 has been shown to be the more potent mitogen.[37] A healing rotator cuff tear model in rabbits showed that the peak expression of FGF-2 was on days 7 and 9, which suggests that it is likely involved in the early phases of tendon healing.[18]

Work on rat patellar tendon and chicken flexor tendon models has further examined the role of FGF-2 in the early phases of tendon healing.[38,39] By injecting various doses of FGF-2 into a rat patellar tendon defect, Chan and colleagues[38] showed that there was a dose-dependent increase in fibroblast proliferation and type III collagen expression 7 days after injection.

Using a chicken digital flexor tendon repair model, Tang and colleagues[39] injected FGF-2 via an adeno-associated viral vector into the tenorrhaphy site before repair. At all time points (2, 4, and 8 weeks after repair), the FGF-2 group was found to have increased ultimate loads-to-failure when compared with controls.

Looking specifically at the effects of FGF-2 on rotator cuff healing, Ide and colleagues[37] applied FGF-2 in a fibrin sealant to repaired supraspinatus tendons in a rat model.

Although this was a pilot study with only 12 animals, the group with locally applied FGF-2 had significantly higher tendon-to-bone insertion maturing scores and ultimate load-to-failure than the control group with fibrin sealant alone at the 2-week time point after repair. At 4 and 6 weeks after repair, the FGF-2–treated and the control group had similar histologic scores and biomechanical strength. These findings further support the role of FGF-2 in accelerating early tendon-to-bone remodeling, and the late similarities between the groups may be attributed to the rapid healing in the rat model of tendon healing.

In a follow-up study, the same group examined the effects of locally applied FGF-2 in a rat rotator cuff model where the supraspinatus tendon was reconstructed with an acellular dermal matrix.[40] The early 2-week time point after repair showed no difference histologically or biomechanically between the treatment and control groups. At the 6- and 12-week time points the FGF-2 treated group had significantly higher histologic scores and strength compared with the untreated group, providing further support for the role of FGF-2 in accelerating and remodeling the tendon repair site.

THE ROLE OF GROWTH FACTORS IN ROTATOR CUFF TENDON-BONE HEALING

As previously discussed, the influx of inflammatory cells during the early phases of tendon healing is the result of cellular and molecular signaling directed by cytokines such as PDGF and TGF-β.[17] These cytokines are also considered growth factors, as they play a crucial role in cell chemotaxis, proliferation, differentiation, and matrix synthesis within the healing enthesis. Because rotator cuff healing results in reactive scar formation rather than a histologically normal insertion site, addition of these factors offers potential to augment the repair-site biology.

PDGF is a basic protein family composed of 2 subunits, an A and a B chain, that exists in 3 main isoforms (PDGF-AA, PDGF-BB, PDGF-AB). These isoforms function as chemotactic agents for inflammatory cells, and help to increase type I collagen synthesis and induce TGF-β1.[19] PDGF is derived from not only platelets but also other cell types, including smooth muscle. The homodimer PDGF-BB isoform has been the subject of most research because it stimulates both matrix synthesis and cell division.[33,41] Work by Kobayashi and colleagues[18] on growth-factor expression during the early healing of the supraspinatus tendon in New Zealand white rabbits showed that the highest concentration of PDGF-BB occurred between days 7 and 14. This period coincides with the terminal part of the inflammatory phase of tendon healing and the early part of the repair phase.

Several studies have examined the role of PDGF as a mitogenic and chemotactic cytokine that can enhance tendon and ligament healing. When used in the treatment of both rat and rabbit knee medial collateral ligament (MCL) rupture models, PDGF was shown to improve the structural and mechanical properties of the femoral-MCL-tibial complexes.[42,43]

In a canine flexor tendon healing model, PDGF-BB delivery was shown to not only accelerate healing but also to increase cell proliferation and matrix remodeling.[44] As a result, the functional properties such as range of motion were improved in the repaired intrasynovial flexor tendons treated with sustained delivery of PDGF-BB. The tensile properties, however, showed no significant difference between the PDGF-BB–treated and control groups. Suboptimal dosing or release kinetics of the PDGF-BB delivery system was postulated to be potential cause for this failure to improve.

Looking specifically at PDGF and rotator cuff healing, Uggen and colleagues[45] showed restoration of normal crimp patterning and collagen-bundle alignment in a rat rotator cuff repair model with delivery of cells expressing PDGF-BB on a polyglycolic acid (PGA) scaffold, compared with controls. As a follow-up study, the same group examined the effects of recombinant human PDGF-BB–coated sutures on rotator cuff healing in a sheep model.[41] This study showed enhanced histologic scores of the treatment group in comparison with controls at short-term follow-up of 6 weeks; however, there was no significant difference between the groups in terms of ultimate load-to-failure. A similar study used an interpositional graft composed of recombinant human PDGF-BB (rhPDGF-BB) and a type I collagen matrix implanted in an ovine model for rotator cuff repair.[46] At 12 weeks after repair, the interpositional graft at low and medium dosages of rhPDGF-BB (75 and 150 µg) had improved biomechanical strength and anatomic appearance compared with the control group and the 500-µg rhPDGF-BB group. These studies highlight again the importance of PDGF-dependent dosing, timing, and delivery methods. Although the exact answer still remains unclear, PDGF augmentation holds promise for augmenting tendon-to-bone healing.

TGF-β is a family of cytokines that includes 3 isoforms (TGF-β1, -2, and -3). Although this superfamily is responsible for numerous physiologic effects, they are of particular interest in biological augmentation, as they are thought to have important roles in tendon and ligament formation through cellular proliferation, differentiation, and matrix synthesis.[33] Of the 3 isoforms, TGF-β3 holds the most promise to enhance the local microenvironment of the rotator cuff repair site because its high expression during fetal wound and tendon healing correlates with no formation of scar tissue.[47] By contrast, postnatal wound healing is characterized by extensive scar formation, with high levels of expression of TGF-β1 and TGF-β2 and low expression of TGF-β3. Because TGF-β3 is not present within the adult healing environment, its exogenous application could potentially promote a regenerative healing process at the tendon-to-bone insertion site.

With this in mind, 3 recent studies have specifically examined the use of TGF-β3 in a rat rotator cuff model.[47–49] The first study by Kim and colleagues[48] used an osmotic pump delivery system to specifically look at the role of TGF-β1 and TGF-β3 at the healing tendon-to-bone insertion of repaired rat supraspinatus tendons. The TGF-β1 group showed increased type III collagen production compared with control shoulders, which is consistent with a scar-mediated healing response. There was also a noted trend toward reduced mechanical properties within this group. By contrast, the TGF-β3 group showed no differences compared with the paired control. While these results further support the TGF-β1 mediated reparative healing response, the lack of improved histologic or biomechanical outcomes in the TGF-β3 group could potentially be attributed to the delivery system used. A subsequent study by the same group using a heparin/fibrin-based delivery system of TGF-β3 to the healing tendon-to-bone insertion demonstrated accelerated healing with increased inflammation, cellularity, vascularity, and cell proliferation at the early time points.[47] In addition, there were significant improvements in structural properties at 28 days and in material properties at 56 days after repair, compared with controls. These findings suggest that TGF-β3 can enhance tendon-to-bone healing in vivo in a rat model.

A study in the authors' laboratory examined the delivery of TGF-β3 in an injectable calcium-phosphate (Ca-P) matrix to the healing tendon-bone interface of repaired rat supraspinatus tendons.[49] The authors found new bone formation, increased fibrocartilage, and improved collagen organization, with augmentation of the tendon-bone repair site with the osteoconductive Ca-P matrix alone in the early postoperative period. With the addition of TGF-β3 to the Ca-P matrix, there was a significant improvement in strength at the repair site 4 weeks postoperatively and a more favorable collagen type I/III ratio, which reflects more mature healing. These results provide further support for the potential of TGF-β3 to improve tendon healing after repair, although future studies are needed to optimize the delivery and dosing as well as to examine the effects of multiple growth factors on the healing process.

PLATELET-RICH PLASMA IN ROTATOR CUFF SURGERY

Many of the growth factors/cytokines involved within the healing response upregulate expression and potentiate the effects of other factors within the cascade of events for repair at the tendon-to-bone insertion. PDGF-BB, for example, has been shown to increase the expression of VEGF in mural cells and in turn induce an angiogenic response by targeting endothelial cells.[50] When combined with IGF-1, PDGF has been shown to work synergistically and positively influence tendon and ligament healing through cell proliferation, differentiation, and matrix formation.[33] In addition, FGF-2 induces the gene expression of TGF-β, which helps to initiate bone ingrowth at the healing enthesis.[37] Because multiple growth factors/cytokines are involved within the various stages of tissue healing, it is reasonable to assume that delivery of these different bioactive factors together could augment healing. Platelet-rich plasma (PRP), which is an autologous concentration of platelets and growth factors that includes PDGF, VEGF, TGF-β, FGF-2, and IGF-1, has therefore become popular as a potential augmentation for tendon healing.

The increased concentration and release of these factors within PRP can potentially enhance the recruitment and proliferation of tenocytes, stem cells, and endothelial cells. Previous animal studies have shown PRP to enhance Achilles tendon stiffness and force to failure in a rat model, and to result in increased vascularity and better tissue organization in rabbit Achilles tendons.[51,52] In human studies, the operative management of Achilles tendon ruptures combined with the application of autologous PRP showed enhanced healing and functional recovery in comparison with matched controls.[53] These results can be contrasted with a recent randomized controlled trial to treat Achilles tendon ruptures with PRP performed by Sánchez and colleagues,[53] in which no beneficial effect on Achilles tendon healing after rupture could be correlated to the application of PRP. These findings highlight the possibility that the effects of PRP could depend on the mechanical loading characteristics of the healing tendon.

Looking specifically at the rotator cuff, several recent studies have examined the use of PRP augmentation at the repair site.[54–59] A prospective level II cohort study out of Seoul, Korea demonstrated that PRP application during arthroscopic rotator cuff repair did not accelerate recovery with respect to pain, range of motion, strength, functional scores, or overall satisfaction when compared with controls at any follow-up time point.[54] The investigators did, however, note a reduced retear rate in the PRP group compared with the control group, but this difference did not reach statistical significance. In a similar case-control study performed by Barber and colleagues,[56] the clinical outcome scores showed no difference between the PRP-augmented arthroscopic rotator cuff repair group and the control group. This study did find, interestingly, that the observed incidence of retears on magnetic resonance imaging was significantly lower in the PRP group than in the control repairs. Of note, a total of 3 and 2 PRP fibrin gels were used in each study, respectively. A similar cohort study performed by Bergeson and colleagues[55] showed no improvement in terms of retear rates or functional outcomes in the PRP-augmented repair group compared with controls. Two platelet-rich fibrin matrix (PRFM) clots were inserted into the repair site in this study.

Two other recent level I randomized control trials examined the effects of PRP augmentation on arthroscopic rotator cuff repairs, with somewhat conflicting results.[57,58] The first, by Randelli and colleagues,[58] showed that local application of PRP resulted in significantly lower pain scores than for the control group within the first postoperative month, but no differences were noted at 3, 6, and 12 months postoperatively. In terms of clinical outcomes, all scores were significantly improved in the PRP group compared with controls (Constant, Strength in External Rotation–modified UCLA, Simple Shoulder Test) at 3 months after surgery. There were no differences noted, however, between the PRP and control groups at 6, 12, and 24 months. The results of this study showed that PRP could have a positive influence on early tendon healing after repair. By contrast, a similar randomized controlled trial by Castricini and colleagues[57] demonstrated that PRP augmentation to the repair site did not improve structural or functional outcomes in comparison with controls.

A randomized controlled study from the authors' institution further supported the work of Castricini and questioned the early healing benefits of PRP by showing no differences between repairs augmented with PRFM and the control group in terms of vascularity and clinical outcomes (American Shoulder and Elbow Surgeons and L'Insalata scores).[59] In addition, the authors found that 67% of the repairs in the PRFM group were intact compared with 81% of the repairs in the control group, which suggests that PRFM may in fact be detrimental to tendon healing in the rotator cuff. From these studies involving PRP, it can be seen that more research and randomized trials are needed to examine why PRP use may improve tendon healing in certain areas and not in others.

CELL-BASED APPROACHES TO AUGMENT TENDON HEALING

As already discussed, the gradations within the mature enthesis that make up the natural rotator cuff tendon-to-bone insertion are not regenerated after a repair. Cytokines generally improve the structural properties of the repair site by increasing formation of new tissue. However, this is typically fibrovascular scar tissue rather than normal insertion site structure and composition, and thus the material properties of healing tissue are not improved. This fact suggests that cytokines still do not provide the cellular and molecular signals to induce true tissue regeneration, which has led the authors to hypothesize that cytokines may need to be combined with undifferentiated cells to improve healing.

Mesenchymal stem cells (MSCs) are characterized by their unique ability to self-renew and differentiate into several different cell lines including osteocytes, chondrocytes, tenocytes, and adipocytes. Factors involved within the specific pathway for MSC differentiation into tenocytes include scleraxis, BMPs, TGF-β3, prostaglandin E$_2$, and mechanical load.[60]

Cell-based approaches may act in one of 3 ways: (1) direct participation in the repair response, (2) a paracrine effect by stimulation of local or distant cells, and (3) anti-inflammatory and/or immunomodulatory effects. Transplanted cells may aid in tendon-to-bone healing, tendon-to-tendon healing, and potentially reversing muscle atrophy and fatty infiltration. The only available autologous cell source at this time are stromal cells isolated from bone marrow, although techniques are now being developed to isolate stromal cells from adipose tissue as well. In the future it may be possible to use induced pluripotent cells or embryonic stem cells to improve healing, as less differentiated and/or more pluripotent cells such as these may hold great promise for improving the healing process.

Mazzocca and colleagues[61] examined the potential to harvest marrow stromal cells from the proximal humerus. These investigators reported that cells isolated from bone marrow aspirated from suture anchor holes in the greater tuberosity at the time of rotator cuff repair were positive for stromal cell markers and had osteogenic potential. This finding demonstrated the possibility of isolating and concentrating local cells at the time of rotator cuff repair. The potential for cell-based approaches to improve healing is also demonstrated by a recent study that reported positive results using laboratory-expanded, skin-derived fibroblasts suspended in autologous plasma to treat Achilles tendonosis. The cells were injected under ultrasound guidance, with significant improvements reported on standardized outcome scales. However, there was no information provided about the appearance of the treated tendons on follow-up ultrasound imaging.[62]

The use of MSCs to enhance tendon regeneration has been examined in multiple animal models of tendon healing. Looking specifically at the rotator cuff in a rat model, work in the authors' laboratory has shown that the use of bone marrow–derived MSCs alone did not improve the histologic or biomechanical properties of the tendon attachment site,[63] suggesting that additional differentiation factors may need to be combined with this cell-based therapy to be effective. Knowledge of the biological signaling events that lead to the formation of the natural enthesis suggests candidate molecules that could be used in combination with MSCs to augment the repair site.

Scleraxis (Scx) is a helix-loop-helix transcription factor that has been found to be necessary for tenogenesis and is important within the developing enthesis.[64] It has been detected within the early phases of mesoderm formation, and in the developing somite it has been found to help define the zone between sclerotomal and myotomal cells.[65] In addition, Scx was found to remain present during the formation of the tendon proper along with the tendon-bone insertion sites. With this concept in mind, a recent study sought to examine the ability of Scx to direct and optimize the differentiation of MSCs during the rotator cuff healing process at the repair site.[65] Using a rat model, bone marrow–derived MSCs were transduced with adenoviral-mediated scleraxis (Ad-Scx) and applied to the tendon-to-bone insertion site after rotator cuff repair. Compared with controls, the Ad-Scx–transduced MSC group had greater stiffness and stress to failure at 2 and 4 weeks after repair and a significantly increased load-to-failure at 4 weeks after repair. Although there were no histologic differences between the Ad-Scx and control groups at 2 weeks after repair, the insertion site of the Ad-Scx group had more fibrocartilage that more closely resembled the native tendon-bone insertion site. This study highlights the potential use of Scx as an augmentation to improve healing of the rotator cuff insertion site after a repair. Further studies still need to be done, however, to fully delineate the signaling mechanism of Scx as well as to investigate its efficacy in larger animal models.

Similar to Scx, BMPs have been shown to be mediators of bone, tendon, and cartilage formation. While the BMPs exist as a group of factors within the TGF-β superfamily, BMP-12, BMP-13, and BMP-14 specifically have each been shown to promote the formation of new tendon when injected ectopically in rats, suggesting that they may be among the key factors that induce tenocyte differentiation.[66,67] In addition, BMP-12, BMP-13, and BMP-14 are unable to induce markers of osteoblastic differentiation such as alkaline phosphatase and osteocalcin in stem cells. Instead, these BMPs seem to drive cells toward tenocyte differentiation. Among these 3, BMP-13 has been shown to be the most potent tenogenic factor.[68,69]

In both rat and rabbit Achilles tendon rupture models, direct injection of each of these 3 proteins increased the tensile strength of the reparative tendon that formed in the defects.[70,71] Within chicken and rabbit flexor-tendon-laceration models, similar effects on tensile strength have been observed.[72–74] Additional studies done at the University of Chicago have demonstrated that recombinant adenoviruses expressing BMP-13 have an efficient dose-dependent transgene expression in rabbit flexor tendons, and that BMP-14 gene therapy increased tendon tensile strength in a rat model of Achilles tendon injury.[75,76] These findings all suggest that BMPs delivered via an adenoviral vector could be used to biologically stimulate and augment tendon repairs.

Looking specifically at the rotator cuff, Seeherman and colleagues[9] used a sheep rotator cuff repair model to examine the healing effects of recombinant human BMP-12 (rhBMP-12) delivered in several carriers.[9] At the final time point of 8 weeks, there was an increase in glycosaminoglycan content and reestablishment of collagen fiber continuity at the bone-tendon interface within the rhBMP-12–treated specimens. Compared with untreated control specimens, the groups treated with rhBMP-12 in collagen and hyaluron sponges were 2.7 and 2.1 times stronger, respectively. The group treated with rhBMP-12 in a hyaluronan paste, however, had similar biomechanical strength to that of the untreated control group. This study demonstrates not only the potential utility of rhBMP-12 in augmenting rotator cuff healing but also the need for an effective delivery vehicle of the growth factor itself.

Another recent study from the authors' laboratory examined the ability of bone marrow–derived MSCs transduced with adenoviral-mediated gene transfer of human BMP-13 (Ad-BMP-13) to improve rotator cuff healing in a rat model.[77] At both the 2- and 4-week time points after repair, there were no differences in new cartilage formation, collagen fiber organization, or biomechanical strength at the repair site between the Ad-BMP-13 group and the untransduced MSC group. These results highlight the poor understanding of the complex signaling events required to regenerate the tendon-to-bone insertion site and that augmentation with a solitary growth factor may not be enough.

ANABOLIC-ANDROGENIC STEROIDS IN TENDON HEALING

Anabolic-androgenic steroids (AASs) are manufactured synthetic derivatives of the hormone testosterone that act on androgenic receptors to exert their positive anabolic effects. By acting at supraphysiologic doses, they have been shown to increase muscle size, muscle strength, collagen synthesis, and bone mineral density.[78] A Swedish study examined the effects of low-dose AASs on the functional outcomes of elderly women after hip fracture surgery, in comparison with vitamin D and calcium or with calcium alone, for 1 year. At final follow-up, the anabolic group had significantly improved speed of gait, Harris hip scores, muscle volume, and bone mineral density.[79]

In relation to tendon injury, AAS use has been associated with tendon rupture by potentially causing a reversible change within the tendon collagen structure that results in a stiffer and less elastic tendon.[78,80] Despite the fact that AAS-induced muscle hypertrophy may make the tendon-to-bone insertion a weak link, experimental studies have suggested a benefit derived from the use of anabolic steroids in rotator cuff tendon healing.[81,82] Using an in vitro rotator cuff model, Triantafillopoulos and colleagues[81] investigated the effects of nandrolone decanoate, a testosterone derivative, and mechanical load on human supraspinatus tenocytes. The load/steroid group had the greatest ultimate stress/strain and a more organized actin cytoskeleton, with increased collagen remodeling. In addition, it was noted that this group also had increased MMP-3 levels. Taken together, these results suggest that steroid use and mechanical load may enhance rotator cuff healing and collagen matrix remodeling in vitro.

More recently, a study by Gerber and colleagues[82] examined the use of anabolic steroids on muscular changes in a rabbit model with chronic rotator cuff tears. Administration of nandrolone decanoate at supramaximal doses was found to prevent fatty infiltration of the supraspinatus muscle and reduce the functional muscle impairment caused by myotendinous retraction.

While these findings suggest a way to prevent muscle deterioration after a tendon tear, care must be taken to recognize the potential side effects of AASs. Within this study, 2 rabbits in the systemic steroid group had to be excluded because of wound infections. It is not known if the steroid application was responsible for the infection; however, the long-term health risk of anabolic steroids at both therapeutic and chronic supraphysiologic doses is unknown. Excessive steroid use has been related to adverse liver and cardiovascular effects. Another global problem with AAS use is that that they are considered performance-enhancing drugs and their use is banned in athletic competitions. Further studies are needed to examine the potential beneficial and adverse effects of AAS augmentation on the healing tendon.

BIOMIMETIC SCAFFOLDS

As previously discussed, the fibrovascular scar that is formed at the tendon-bone repair site is notably weaker than the native enthesis and is therefore at increased risk for failure.[83] To help augment or stimulate a more regenerative healing response with less scar formation, the previous sections have examined delivery of various growth factors or AAS to the repair site. However, problems still remain regarding the delivery methods of these factors, optimal dosing, and potential optimal combinations. From this perspective, new strategies in tissue engineering have evolved that have focused on a biomimetic scaffold that has the ability to achieve a functional integration within the host environment.[84] The ideal scaffold would be multiphased to restore the tissue organization and mechanical properties of the native insertion site. A key feature is that these phases must be interconnected to promote regeneration of the bone-tendon interface.

Current approaches for ideal scaffold design have focused on nanofiber-based structures because their fabrication can incorporate matrix anisotropy as well as region-dependent changes.[13] Although a full review of the various nanofiber scaffold designs is beyond the scope of this article, a highlight of recent applications for tendon tissue engineering is examined here.

Recently, Zhang and colleagues[13] constructed a biphasic scaffold consisting of polylactide-co-glycolide (PLGA) nanofibers as the first phase, and a composite of PLGA nanofibers and hydroxyapatite nanoparticles as the second phase. The main purpose of this design was to stimulate regeneration of both the nonmineralized and mineralized fibrocartilage regions of the enthesis and to promote osteointegration with the PLGA-hydroxyapatite nanofibers. The group then tested this scaffold in an in vivo Lewis rat rotator cuff model. Their findings showed that the biphasic scaffold promoted the formation of a continuous noncalcified and calcified matrix region, whereas only fibrovascular scar was observed in the control group. Further studies have examined controlling scaffold mineral distribution as another potential approach to promote regenerative healing at the tendon-to-bone insertion site.[85,86]

The use of nanotechnology-based designs to create biomimetic scaffolds holds promise as an augmentation for connective tissue repair. Future research still needs to be done, however, to fully examine and understand the exact mechanisms and signaling events that lead to the formation of the graded structures between the different types of connective tissue at the enthesis.[13] An understanding of the developmental biology at the tendon-bone insertion site will directly affect scaffold design and potentially lead to the incorporation of growth factors or other signaling molecules within these structures.

THE FUTURE

While gene therapy has been examined as a potential strategy for growth factor delivery, the next frontier involves the use of small interfering RNA (siRNA) as a means to modulate gene expression.[87] Effective delivery of siRNA can be accomplished through viral-mediated or nonviral-mediated vector-based delivery systems. The barriers to siRNA delivery, however, depend on the target organs and the route of administration.

Two recent studies have examined siRNA therapy as it relates to osteoarthritis and aseptic loosening in total joint implants.[88,89] In the first study, Li and colleagues[88] used RNA interference technology to downregulate the transcription factor c-maf and subsequently reduce the expression of MMP-13. Because the level of MMP-13 is elevated in pathologic conditions leading to destruction of cartilage tissue, regulation of its expression by c-maf may help to control the onset and progression of osteoarthritis. A second study by Peng and colleagues[89] examined the use of siRNA targeting tumor necrosis factor α (TNF-α) as a means to reduce wear debris–provoked inflammation. Using a lentiviral-mediated TNF-α siRNA in a murine air-pouch model, the investigators showed that the locally delivered siRNA was able to block TNF-α expression on both mRNA and protein levels. In addition, it was noted that expression of the inflammatory mediators interleukin-1 and interleukin-6 were downregulated as a result of lentivirus-mediated TNF-α siRNA.

Regarding tissue engineering, siRNA-based therapies have the potential to regulate the expression of the various factors that enhance the healing process. A study by Cheema and colleagues[90] demonstrated that siRNA-mediated downregulation of guanine nucleotide–binding protein α-stimulating activity polypeptide 1 (GNAS1) led to enhanced expression of core-binding factor α1 (Cbfα1), also known as Runx2. Cbfα1 is a transcriptional regulator of both osteoblast differentiation and function. This increased expression of CBFα1 could potentially result in regulated osteogenic differentiation of MSCs because of the enhanced production of bone-differentiating genes.

Although no current clinical trials using siRNA-based therapies for musculoskeletal conditions are being conducted, its application holds promise as a method to augment bone-to-tendon healing. The future directions will include optimal delivery methods and gene targets. However, SiRNA therapy is not without risk, as safety concerns do exist with regard to the use of viral vectors in gene therapy. Further research is needed to determine whether nonviral gene transfer is an effective and safer alternative to viral-based therapies.

SUMMARY

The rotator cuff enthesis is not reestablished after a rotator cuff repair. Instead, a scar-mediated healing response occurs at the tendon-bone interface, which is notably weaker than the native enthesis and thus more prone to failure. Biological augmentation through growth factors, AASs, biomimetic scaffolds, or siRNA therapy has the potential to enhance the healing response. The ultimate key, however, is in determining which of these enables a more regenerative healing response of the native tissue rather than enhanced production of scar tissue. In addition, the optimal combination of factors, dosing, and delivery methods remains to be clearly elucidated. Biological augmentation and tissue engineering for tendon healing remains promising, but much work still needs to be done.

REFERENCES

1. Boileau P, Brassart N, Watkinson DJ, et al. Arthroscopic repair of full-thickness tears of the supraspinatus: does the tendon really heal? J Bone Joint Surg Am 2005;87(6):1229–40.
2. Rodeo S, Potter H, Kawamura S, et al. Biologic augmentation of rotator cuff tendon-healing with use of a mixture of osteoinductive growth factors. J Bone Joint Surg Am 2007;89(11):2485–97.
3. Galatz LM, Ball CM, Teefey SA, et al. The outcome and repair integrity of completely arthroscopically repaired large and massive rotator cuff tears. J Bone Joint Surg Am 2004;86-A(2):219–24.
4. Gamradt SC, Rodeo SA, Warren RF. Platelet rich plasma in rotator cuff repair. Tech Orthop 2007;22(1):26–33. http://dx.doi.org/10.1097/1001.bto.0000261868. 0000203232.dd.
5. Harryman DT 2nd, Mack LA, Wang KY, et al. Repairs of the rotator cuff. Correlation of functional results with integrity of the cuff. J Bone Joint Surg Am 1991; 73(7):982–9.
6. Gerber C, Fuchs B, Hodler J. The results of repair of massive tears of the rotator cuff. J Bone Joint Surg Am 2000;82(4):505–15.
7. Lafosse L, Brozska R, Toussaint B, et al. The outcome and structural integrity of arthroscopic rotator cuff repair with use of the double-row suture anchor technique. J Bone Joint Surg Am 2007;89(7):1533–41.
8. Dines JS, Grande DA, Dines DM. Tissue engineering and rotator cuff tendon healing. J Shoulder Elbow Surg 2007;16(Suppl 5):S204–7.
9. Seeherman H, Archambault J, Rodeo S, et al. rhBMP-12 accelerates healing of rotator cuff repairs in a sheep model. J Bone Joint Surg Am 2008;90(10):2206–19.
10. Nho SJ, Delos D, Yadav H, et al. Biomechanical and biologic augmentation for the treatment of massive rotator cuff tears. Am J Sports Med 2010;38(3):619–29.
11. Gulotta LV, Rodeo SA. Growth factors for rotator cuff repair. Clin Sports Med 2009; 28(1):13–23.

12. Galatz L, Rothermich S, VanderPloeg K, et al. Development of the supraspinatus tendon-to-bone insertion: localized expression of extracellular matrix and growth factor genes. J Orthop Res 2007;25(12):1621–8.
13. Zhang X, Bogdanowicz D, Erisken C, et al. Biomimetic scaffold design for functional and integrative tendon repair. J Shoulder Elbow Surg 2012;21(2):266–77.
14. Carpenter J, Thomopoulos S, Flanagan C, et al. Rotator cuff defect healing: a biomechanical and histologic analysis in an animal model. J Shoulder Elbow Surg 1998;7(6):599–605.
15. Galatz LM, Sandell LJ, Rothermich SY, et al. Characteristics of the rat supraspinatus tendon during tendon-to-bone healing after acute injury. J Orthop Res 2006;24(3):541–50.
16. Edwards SL, Lynch TS, Saltzman MD, et al. Biologic and pharmacologic augmentation of rotator cuff repairs. J Am Acad Orthop Surg 2011;19(10):583–9.
17. Rodeo S. Biologic augmentation of rotator cuff tendon repair. J Shoulder Elbow Surg 2007;16(Suppl 5):S191–7.
18. Kobayashi M, Itoi E, Minagawa H, et al. Expression of growth factors in the early phase of supraspinatus tendon healing in rabbits. J Shoulder Elbow Surg 2006; 15(3):371–7.
19. Würgler-Hauri CC, Dourte LM, Baradet TC, et al. Temporal expression of 8 growth factors in tendon-to-bone healing in a rat supraspinatus model. J Shoulder Elbow Surg 2007;16(Suppl 5):S198–203.
20. Pasternak B, Aspenberg P. Metalloproteinases and their inhibitors—diagnostic and therapeutic opportunities in orthopedics. Acta Orthop 2009;80(6):693–703.
21. Pearce WH, Shively VP. Abdominal aortic aneurysm as a complex multifactorial disease: interactions of polymorphisms of inflammatory genes, features of autoimmunity, and current status of MMPs. Ann N Y Acad Sci 2006;1085: 117–32.
22. Bedi A, Fox AJS, Kovacevic D, et al. Doxycycline-mediated inhibition of matrix metalloproteinases improves healing after rotator cuff repair. Am J Sports Med 2010;38(2):308–17.
23. Shindle MK, Chen CC, Robertson C, et al. Full-thickness supraspinatus tears are associated with more synovial inflammation and tissue degeneration than partial-thickness tears. J Shoulder Elbow Surg 2001;20(6):917–27.
24. Pasternak B, Schepull T, Eliasson P, et al. Elevation of systemic matrix metalloproteinases 2 and 7 and tissue inhibitor of metalloproteinase 2 in patients with a history of Achilles tendon rupture: pilot study. Br J Sports Med 2010;44(9): 669–72.
25. Lo IK, Marchuk LL, Hollinshead R, et al. Matrix metalloproteinase and tissue inhibitor of matrix metalloproteinase mRNA levels are specifically altered in torn rotator cuff tendons. Am J Sports Med 2004;32(5):1223–9.
26. Yoshihara Y, Hamada K, Nakajima T, et al. Biochemical markers in the synovial fluid of glenohumeral joints from patients with rotator cuff tear. J Orthop Res 2001;19(4):573–9.
27. McDowell CL, Marqueen TJ, Yager D, et al. Characterization of the tensile properties and histologic/biochemical changes in normal chicken tendon at the site of suture insertion. J Hand Surg 2002;27(4):605–14.
28. Pasternak B, Missios A, Askendal A, et al. Doxycycline-coated sutures improve the suture-holding capacity of the rat Achilles tendon. Acta Othop 2007;78(5): 680–6.
29. Brooks CH, Revell WJ, Heatley FW. A quantitative histological study of the vascularity of the rotator cuff tendon. J Bone Joint Surg Br 1992;74(1):151–3.

30. Cadet ER, Adler RS, Gallo RA, et al. Contrast-enhanced ultrasound characterization of the vascularity of the repaired rotator cuff tendon: short-term and intermediate-term follow-up. J Shoulder Elbow Surg 2012;21(5):597–603.
31. Fealy S, Adler RS, Drakos MC, et al. Patterns of vascular and anatomical response after rotator cuff repair. Am J Sports Med 2006;34(1):120–7.
32. Gamradt SC, Gallo RA, Adler RS, et al. Vascularity of the supraspinatus tendon three months after repair: characterization using contrast-enhanced ultrasound. J Shoulder Elbow Surg 2010;19(1):73–80.
33. Oliva F, Via AG, Maffulli N. Role of growth factors in rotator cuff healing. Sports Med Arthrosc 2011;19(3):218–26.
34. Bidder M, Towler DA, Gelberman RH, et al. Expression of mRNA for vascular endothelial growth factor at the repair site of healing canine flexor tendon. J Orthop Res 2000;18(2):247–52.
35. Zhang F, Liu H, Stile F, et al. Effect of vascular endothelial growth factor on rat Achilles tendon healing. Plast Reconstr Surg 2003;112(6):1613–9.
36. Yoshikawa T, Tohyama H, Katsura T, et al. Effects of local administration of vascular endothelial growth factor on mechanical characteristics of the semitendinosus tendon graft after anterior cruciate ligament reconstruction in sheep. Am J Sports Med 2006;34(12):1918–25.
37. Ide J, Kikukawa K, Hirose J, et al. The effect of a local application of fibroblast growth factor-2 on tendon-to-bone remodeling in rats with acute injury and repair of the supraspinatus tendon. J Shoulder Elbow Surg 2009;18(3):391–8.
38. Chan BP, Fu S, Qin L, et al. Effects of basic fibroblast growth factor (bFGF) on early stages of tendon healing: a rat patellar tendon model. Acta Orthop Scand 2000;71(5):513–8.
39. Tang JB, Cao Y, Zhu B, et al. Adeno-associated virus-2-mediated bFGF gene transfer to digital flexor tendons significantly increases healing strength. An in vivo study. J Bone Joint Surg Am 2008;90(5):1078–89.
40. Ide J, Kikukawa K, Hirose J, et al. The effects of fibroblast growth factor-2 on rotator cuff reconstruction with acellular dermal matrix grafts. Arthroscopy 2009;25(6):608–16.
41. Uggen C, Dines J, McGarry M, et al. The effect of recombinant human platelet-derived growth factor bb-coated sutures on rotator cuff healing in a sheep model. Arthroscopy 2010;26(11):1456–62.
42. Letson AK, Dahners LE. The effect of combinations of growth factors on ligament healing. Clin Orthop Relat Res 1994;(308):207–12.
43. Hildebrand KA, Woo SL, Smith DW, et al. The effects of platelet-derived growth factor-BB on healing of the rabbit medial collateral ligament. An in vivo study. Am J Sports Med 1998;26(4):549–54.
44. Thomopoulos S, Zaegel M, Das R, et al. PDGF-BB released in tendon repair using a novel delivery system promotes cell proliferation and collagen remodeling. J Orthop Res 2007;25(10):1358–68.
45. Uggen JC, Dines J, Uggen CW, et al. Tendon gene therapy modulates the local repair environment in the shoulder. J Am Osteopath Assoc 2005;105(1):20–1.
46. Hee CK, Dines JS, Dines DM, et al. Augmentation of a rotator cuff suture repair using rhPDGF-BB and a type I bovine collagen matrix in an ovine model. Am J Sports Med 2011;39(8):1630–9.
47. Manning CN, Kim HM, Sakiyama-Elbert S, et al. Sustained delivery of transforming growth factor beta three enhances tendon-to-bone healing in a rat model. J Orthop Res 2011;29(7):1099–105.

48. Kim HM, Galatz LM, Das R, et al. The role of transforming growth factor beta isoforms in tendon-to-bone healing. Connect Tissue Res 2011;52(2):87–98.
49. Kovacevic D, Fox AJ, Bedi A, et al. Calcium-phosphate matrix with or without TGF-beta3 improves tendon-bone healing after rotator cuff repair. Am J Sports Med 2011;39(4):811–9.
50. Hollinger J, Hart C, Hirsch S, et al. Recombinant human platelet-derived growth factor: biology and clinical applications. J Bone Joint Surg Am 2008;90(Suppl 1): 48–54.
51. Aspenberg P, Virchenko O. Platelet concentrate injection improves Achilles tendon repair in rats. Acta Orthop Scand 2004;75(1):93–9.
52. Lyras DN, Kazakos K, Verettas D, et al. The influence of platelet-rich plasma on angiogenesis during the early phase of tendon healing. Foot Ankle Int 2009; 30(11):1101–6.
53. Sánchez M, Anitua E, Azofra J, et al. Comparison of surgically repaired Achilles tendon tears using platelet-rich fibrin matrices. Am J Sports Med 2007;35(2): 245–51.
54. Jo CH, Kim JE, Yoon KS, et al. Does platelet-rich plasma accelerate recovery after rotator cuff repair? A prospective cohort study. Am J Sports Med 2011; 39(10):2082–90.
55. Bergeson AG, Tashjian RZ, Greis PE, et al. Effects of platelet-rich fibrin matrix on repair integrity of at-risk rotator cuff tears. Am J Sports Med 2012;40(2): 286–93.
56. Barber FA, Hrnack SA, Snyder SJ, et al. Rotator cuff repair healing influenced by platelet-rich plasma construct augmentation. Arthroscopy 2011;27(8):1029–35.
57. Castricini R, Longo UG, De Benedetto M, et al. Platelet-rich plasma augmentation for arthroscopic rotator cuff repair: a randomized controlled trial. Am J Sports Med 2011;39(2):258–65.
58. Randelli P, Arrigoni P, Ragone V, et al. Platelet rich plasma in arthroscopic rotator cuff repair: a prospective RCT study, 2-year follow-up. J Shoulder Elbow Surg 2011;20(4):518–28.
59. Rodeo SA, Delos D, Williams RJ, et al. The effect of platelet-rich fibrin matrix on rotator cuff tendon healing: a prospective randomized clinical study. Presented at the American Shoulder and Elbow Surgeons 2010 Closed Meeting, Scottsdale (AZ). 2012;40(6):1234–41.
60. Gulotta LV, Chaudhury S, Wiznia D. Stem cells for augmenting tendon repair. Stem Cells Int 2012;2012:291431.
61. Mazzocca AD, McCarthy MB, Chowaniec DM, et al. Rapid isolation of human stem cells (connective tissue progenitor cells) from the proximal humerus during arthroscopic rotator cuff surgery. Am J Sports Med 2010;38(7):1438–47.
62. Obaid H, Clarke A, Rosenfeld P, et al. Skin-derived fibroblasts for the treatment of refractory Achilles tendinosis: preliminary short-term results. J Bone Joint Surg Am 2012;94(3):193–200.
63. Gulotta LV, Kovacevic D, Ehteshami JR, et al. Application of bone marrow-derived mesenchymal stem cells in a rotator cuff repair model. Am J Sports Med 2009; 37(11):2126–33.
64. Thomopoulos S, Genin GM, Galatz LM. The development and morphogenesis of the tendon-to-bone insertion—what development can teach us about healing. J Musculoskelet Neuronal Interact 2010;10(1):35–45.
65. Gulotta LV, Kovacevic D, Packer JD, et al. Bone marrow-derived mesenchymal stem cells transduced with scleraxis improve rotator cuff healing in a rat model. Am J Sports Med 2011;39(6):1282–9.

66. Aspenberg P, Forslund C. Enhanced tendon healing with GDF 5 and 6. Acta Orthop Scand 1999;70(1):51–4.
67. Cheng H, Jiang W, Phillips FM, et al. Osteogenic activity of the fourteen types of human bone morphogenetic proteins (BMPs). J Bone Joint Surg Am 2003; 85-A(8):1544–52.
68. Forslund C, Aspenberg P. Tendon healing stimulated by injected CDMP-2. Med Sci Sports Exerc 2001;33(5):685–7.
69. Virchenko O, Fahlgren A, Skoglund B, et al. CDMP-2 injection improves early tendon healing in a rabbit model for surgical repair. Scand J Med Sci Sports 2005;15(4):260–4.
70. Luo J, Sun MH, Kang Q, et al. Gene therapy for bone regeneration. Curr Gene Ther 2005;5(2):167–79.
71. Wolfman NM, Hattersley G, Cox K, et al. Ectopic induction of tendon and ligament in rats by growth and differentiation factors 5, 6, and 7, members of the TGF-beta gene family. J Clin Invest 1997;100(2):321–30.
72. Lou J. In vivo gene transfer into tendon by recombinant adenovirus. Clin Orthop Relat Res 2000;(Suppl 379):S252–5.
73. Lou J, Tu Y, Burns M, et al. BMP-12 gene transfer augmentation of lacerated tendon repair. J Orthop Res 2001;19(6):1199–202.
74. Lou J, Manske PR, Aoki M, et al. Adenovirus-mediated gene transfer into tendon and tendon sheath. J Orthop Res 1996;14(4):513–7.
75. Bolt P, Clerk A, Luu H, et al. BMP-14 gene therapy increases tendon tensile strength in a rat model of Achilles tendon injury. J Bone Joint Surg Am 2007; 89(6):1315–20.
76. Mehta V, Kang Q, Luo J, et al. Characterization of adenovirus-mediated gene transfer in rabbit flexor tendons. J Hand Surg 2005;30(1):136–41.
77. Gulotta LV, Kovacevic D, Packer JD, et al. Adenoviral-mediated gene transfer of human bone morphogenetic protein-13 does not improve rotator cuff healing in a rat model. Am J Sports Med 2011;39(1):180–7.
78. Evans NA. Current concepts in anabolic-androgenic steroids. Am J Sports Med 2004;32(2):534–42.
79. Hedstrom M, Sjoberg K, Brosjo E, et al. Positive effects of anabolic steroids, vitamin D and calcium on muscle mass, bone mineral density and clinical function after a hip fracture. A randomised study of 63 women. J Bone Joint Surg Br 2002;84(4):497–503.
80. Miles JW, Grana WA, Egle D, et al. The effect of anabolic steroids on the biomechanical and histological properties of rat tendon. J Bone Joint Surg Am 1992; 74(3):411–22.
81. Triantafillopoulos IK, Banes AJ, Bowman KF Jr, et al. Nandrolone decanoate and load increase remodeling and strength in human supraspinatus bioartificial tendons. Am J Sports Med 2004;32(4):934–43.
82. Gerber C, Meyer DC, Nuss KM, et al. Anabolic steroids reduce muscle damage caused by rotator cuff tendon release in an experimental study in rabbits. J Bone Joint Surg Am 2011;93(23):2189–95.
83. Smith L, Xia Y, Galatz LM, et al. Tissue engineering strategies for the tendon/ligament-to-bone insertion. Connect Tissue Res 2012;53(2):95–105.
84. Lu HH, Subramony SD, Boushell MK, et al. Tissue engineering strategies for the regeneration of orthopedic interfaces. Ann Biomed Eng 2010;38(6):2142–54.
85. Erisken C, Kalyon DM, Wang H. Functionally graded electrospun polycaprolactone and beta-tricalcium phosphate nanocomposites for tissue engineering applications. Biomaterials 2008;29(30):4065–73.

86. Li X, Xie J, Lipner J, et al. Nanofiber scaffolds with gradations in mineral content for mimicking the tendon-to-bone insertion site. Nano Lett 2009;9(7):2763–8.
87. Shi Q, Zhang XL, Dai KR, et al. siRNA therapy for cancer and non-lethal diseases such as arthritis and osteoporosis. Expert Opin Biol Ther 2011;11(1):5–16.
88. Li T, Xiao J, Wu Z, et al. Transcriptional activation of human MMP-13 gene expression by c-Maf in osteoarthritic chondrocyte. Connect Tissue Res 2010;51(1): 48–54.
89. Peng X, Tao K, Cheng T, et al. Efficient inhibition of wear debris-induced inflammation by locally delivered siRNA. Biochem Biophys Res Commun 2008;377(2): 532–7.
90. Cheema SK, Chen E, Shea LD, et al. Regulation and guidance of cell behavior for tissue regeneration via the siRNA mechanism. Wound Repair Regen 2007;15(3): 286–95.

Outcomes of Rotator Cuff Surgery
What Does the Evidence Tell Us?

Alexander W. Aleem, MD, Robert H. Brophy, MD*

KEYWORDS

- Rotator cuff repair • Shoulder arthroscopy • Rotator cuff tear • Mini-open repair

KEY POINTS

- Rotator cuff tears are a common clinical problem that increases with age from an incidence of 4% in those aged 40 to 60 years to more than 54% in those older than 60 years.[1]
- The purpose of this article is to review the current evidence regarding outcomes of surgical techniques in rotator cuff surgery.
- Future research should be aimed at identifying whether and in whom rotator cuff healing is appropriate to better identify surgical candidates as well as to determine the best surgical repair strategy.

INTRODUCTION

Rotator cuff tears are a common clinical problem that increases with age from an incidence of 4% in those aged 40 to 60 years to more than 54% in those older than 60 years.[1] Symptomatic rotator cuff tears can be successfully treated with nonoperative and operative treatment.[2] Indications for surgical intervention are not widely agreed on as evidenced by the results of a survey of the American Academy of Orthopedic Surgeons' (AAOS) membership.[3] Relevant factors include duration and severity of symptoms, acuity of tear, weakness, size of the tear, and muscle atrophy and fatty infiltration.[2,4] Despite the lack of consistent evidence-based agreement on indications, surgical treatment of the rotator cuff has been used since 1911.[5] The technique has evolved from the open approach used by Dr Codman 100 years ago to first the mini-open technique and subsequently to all arthroscopic techniques, which can be used to treat partial-thickness tears as well as full-thickness tears. The purpose of this article is to review the latest evidence for outcomes from rotator cuff surgery.

Disclosures: None.
Department of Orthopaedic Surgery, Washington University School of Medicine, 14532 South Outer Forty Drive, Chesterfield, MO 63017, USA
* Corresponding author.
E-mail address: brophyr@wudosis.wustl.edu

OPEN SURGERY

Sixty years after Dr Codman's initial description of open rotator cuff surgery in the early twentieth century,[5] Neer[6] ushered in the modern era of rotator cuff surgery with his report on outcomes after the release and repair of torn rotator cuff tendons combined with anterior acromioplasty. He described 5 fundamental principles for open rotator cuff surgery: (1) meticulous repair of the deltoid origin, (2) subacromial decompression with division of the coracoacromial ligament, (3) release of the cuff as needed to obtain freely mobile muscle-tendon units, (4) secure transosseous fixation of the tendon to the greater tuberosity, and (5) closely supervised rehabilitation with early passive motion. Open rotator cuff repair has been shown to result in good to excellent outcomes in terms of functional improvement (75%–95% of patients) and pain relief (85%–100%).[4,7–13]

MINI-OPEN

Because of the concerns about morbidity resulting from taking down the deltoid, Levy and colleagues[14] described an arthroscopic-assisted approach to rotator cuff repair in 1990. The shoulder and rotator cuff could be inspected and prepared (including sub-acromial decompression) without taking down the deltoid. Any intra-articular lesion found during arthroscopy could also be treated. The repair could even be initiated arthroscopically before extending the lateral portal to facilitate mini-open access to complete the repair, typically via transosseous sutures. Limiting the extent of the deltoid exposure both in terms of size and time potentially limits the risk for deltoid injury. Repair of the rotator cuff still adhered to Neer's fundamental principles of release of the cuff to obtain freely mobile units and secure transosseous fixation.

Several studies following Levy's initial description reported good to excellent results in terms of pain relief and functional improvement (85%–95% of patients) in the short-term and long-term follow-up.[14–18] In 1995, Baker and Liu[19] compared open repair with mini-open repair and found equally effective results in terms of pain relief and functional outcomes. They also reported shorter hospital stays and quicker return to activity in the arthroscopic mini-open group versus the open group. Patients with tears larger than 3 cm who had arthroscopic-assisted repair had numerically lower functional outcome scores than those with smaller tears who also received mini-open repair, but the difference was not statistically significant. This trend of poorer outcomes with larger tears is also consistent with results using open techniques.[11]

In a randomized control trial comparing the open technique with the mini-open technique, short-term (3 month) quality-of-life measures were both statistically and clinically improved in the mini-open group compared with the open cohort.[20] There was no difference between the groups in terms of functional outcome measures at the 1- or 2-year follow-up.

The mini-open technique gives surgeons the ability to evaluate the glenohumeral joint and perform subacromial decompressions without needing to take down the deltoid, both of which could not be done with traditional open techniques. Several studies cited a large percentage (60%–75%) of patients who had intra-articular pathologic conditions that would have gone unrecognized with standard open techniques.[16–18] Additionally, decreased trauma to the deltoid theoretically contributes to decreased postoperative pain and allows for more aggressive early postoperative rehabilitation.

ARTHROSCOPIC

As arthroscopic skills and techniques improved, surgeons began to attempt all arthroscopic repairs. The cited advantages of all arthroscopic repairs include small skin incisions, access to the glenohumeral joint for inspection and treatment of intra-articular lesions, and less soft tissue dissection.[21-23] Standard glenohumeral shoulder arthroscopy is performed that addresses and diagnoses intra-articular lesions. The arthroscope is then directed to the subacromial space where the reparability of the tendons is assessed. Subacromial decompression and acromioplasty is performed to allow space for the repair and the fixed tendon. The tendon may require mobilization before repair. The tendons are then repaired typically with sutures from anchors and often with the aid of different accessory portals determined by the location and size of the tear.

The results reported using all arthroscopic repair techniques are similar to those of open and mini-open repairs, with 85% to 95% of patients having improved pain relief and functional outcomes.[21,22] Some studies also found that larger tears (>3 cm) had comparable results to those with small to medium size tears, a departure from other techniques. Advocates for all arthroscopic repairs argue that arthroscopy gives surgeons the ability and flexibility with various portal locations to completely visualize and analyze a tear.[24] Repair can then be optimized based on this complete visualization.

Suture anchors are commonly used during all arthroscopic repairs of cuff tears. They theoretically provide the same fixation strength to bone as a suture looped through transosseous tunnels. Unfortunately, no clinical studies exist directly comparing suture anchors with transosseous tunnels. The technical goal of achieving stable fixation of the tendon to bone seems to be more important than the fixation technique used because equivalent patient outcome results have been reported with techniques using bone tunnels and suture anchors. Therefore, fixation is typically selected based on the surgeon's preference.

Despite the theoretical advantages of all arthroscopic repair in terms of complete visualization of the tear and minimal morbidity, there has been no documented significant difference in patient outcomes when compared with other techniques. Several investigators have compared results for arthroscopic versus mini-open repair with both groups having equivalent results.[25-27] Similar conclusions have also been found when comparing open versus arthroscopic repair.[28,29] No study has compared all 3 described techniques, so it is impossible to state that one technique is better than the others. Given the theoretical advantages of smaller skin incisions, no deltoid detachment, and less soft tissue dissection, arthroscopic techniques continue to gain popularity for the treatment of rotator cuff tears.

SINGLE-ROW VERSUS DOUBLE-ROW REPAIR

As all arthroscopic techniques have become increasingly popular, more investigation into the configuration of fixation has been allocated. Bishop and colleagues[30] noted a high rate of recurrence of tears in arthroscopic repair patients versus open repair, especially in those with large (>3 cm) tears. Similarly, Galatz and colleagues[31] found that 17 out of 18 patients with large (>2 cm) rotator cuff tears had evidence of recurrent defects following repair but had improved pain relief and functional scores. Some studies demonstrate superior outcomes in shoulders with healed cuff tears compared with those with persistent or recurrent tears.[32,33] However, other studies have shown that failure of healing does not necessarily correlate with symptoms.[31]

A single-row method of anchor fixation was used in these studies, meaning that one row of suture anchors is placed in the greater tuberosity on the lateral aspect of the rotator cuff footprint. This method does not completely recreate the native footprint insertion of the supraspinatus tendon on the greater tuberosity but rather spot-welds it, potentially leading to incomplete anatomic healing.[34] This circumstance has lead to the use of a double-row technique in which a second row of suture anchors is placed medially closer to the articular margin and one set of sutures is shared between the two rows acting to compress the rotator cuff on its native footprint in addition to increasing the surface area for healing.[35,36]

Biomechanical and cadaver studies have shown that a double-row repair is superior to single-row repair in terms of fixation strength.[37] Additionally, cadaver studies have shown that double-row repairs restore the supraspinatus footprint closer to its original site.[38] A clinical intraoperative study found that, on average, a single-row repair left 52.7% of the footprint uncovered, whereas double-row repairs provided complete coverage.[39] Systematic reviews support the claim that double-row fixation is biomechanically superior to single-row fixation.[40,41]

Despite the biomechanical advantage, clinical studies comparing patient outcomes following single- versus double-row fixation have been less convincing of any advantage of a double-row technique. Most of the data are retrospective in nature, but there are 3 randomized controlled trials comparing the two methods.[42–44] Wall and colleagues[40] reviewed these studies and 2 nonrandomized prospective clinical trials and found similar equivalence in functional results at the short-term follow-up for single-row versus double-row fixation. There is still a lack of long-term follow-up studies of patient outcomes with double-row repair.

A systematic review performed by Saridakis and Jones[41] found that despite the benefit of structural healing in double-row fixation, there were not any superior clinical outcomes when comparing all comers of rotator cuff repair. However, for patients with large to massive tears (>3 cm), they did find improved functional outcomes. Double-row procedures are technically more difficult, more time consuming, and more expensive compared with single-row repairs. They concluded that double-row fixation has a place for patients that have large tears and/or have higher functional demands and a risk-reward analysis of patient age, functional demands, and quality-of-life issues should be used before deciding which method to use.

More recently, there has been interest in the so-called transosseous-equivalent repair. Park and colleagues[45] originally described this technique in which a medial row of suture anchors is placed with sutures tied in a mattress fashion. The suture limbs are then preserved and bridged over the footprint insertion with distal-lateral interference screw fixation. This repair differs from double-row fixation by not needing a second row of suture anchors and theoretically maximizes tendon-to-bone compression. Biomechanical studies have confirmed that transosseous-equivalent repair provides more contact area and pressure over the footprint compared with double-row fixation[46] as well as equivalent strength compared with traditional open transosseous techniques.[47] Short-term clinical studies have shown favorable results functionally and structurally with outcomes comparable with double-row fixation.[48] Comparative studies to other fixation methods and long-term follow-up studies have yet to be published, but the early evidence of transosseous-equivalent repair is promising.

COLLAGEN AUGMENTATION

Investigators have looked at other ways to optimize the healing of rotator cuff tendon repairs. Given the decreased evidence of radiologic healing and potentially higher retear rate for larger tears, most investigation has focused on augmenting the repair for medium to massive tears. Various collagen allografts and xenografts have been used in other orthopedic settings as scaffolds for tendon healing.[49]

One such xenograft is porcine small intestine submucosa. This type of graft has had success with repair in Achilles tendon ruptures and a canine model of infraspinatus tears as a biologic scaffold for repair.[49] Results in clinical trials for rotator cuff repair have been less clear. A consecutive study of 11 patients who underwent repairs with porcine small intestine submucosa augmentation showed that at 6 months, 10 out of 11 had magnetic resonance imaging (MRI) evidence of re-tear.[42,50] The 11th patient retore at 10 months. Additionally, there was no improvement in preoperative versus postoperative shoulder scores.

Two comparative clinical trials, including one randomized clinical trial, also investigated the efficacy of porcine small intestine submucosa xenograft augmentation.[49,51] Both studies showed worse outcomes in terms of pain and function compared with primary repair alone. A high proportion (20%–30%) of patients in the xenograft group also had hypersensitivity to the grafts that manifested as a severe inflammatory response. Based on these negative results, porcine intestine submucosa is not recommended for augmentation in rotator cuff tear repair.

Various other allografts and xenografts are commercially available and differ from porcine small intestine submucosa in both biologic and mechanical composition. Examples include collagen allograft matrices and porcine dermal xenografts.[52,53] Studies investigating other augmentation graft options show favorable results in terms of patient outcomes and healing. However, these studies are small and generally not well designed, making it difficult to draw conclusions based on their effectiveness.[52,53] These options warrant further investigation and may serve a larger role in the future.

BIOLOGIC AUGMENTATION

Recent investigation has also been dedicated to the biologic side of rotator cuff tendon healing and possible biologic augmentation that may help improve rotator cuff tendon healing. Tendon healing occurs in 3 overlapping stages: inflammatory, fibroblastic, and remodeling.[54] Inflammation occurs within the first week after repair and is characterized by deposition of fibrin and fibronectin by platelets. The platelets secrete various growth factors that recruit macrophages and neutrophils. Macrophages then secrete transforming growth factor–beta1, which promotes scar tissue formation. The fibroblastic stage begins within 48 hours of repair and can last for up to 8 weeks. During this period, fibroblasts produce primarily type III collagen. During the remodeling stage, type III collagen is remodeled into a more organized matrix by type I. The end result is tissue that resembles scar tissue rather than normally composed native tendon.[55–57]

Various animal and histologic studies have been done to investigate the potential of various growth factors as biologic augments. These growth factors include bone morphogenic protein, fibroblast growth factors, and matrix metalloproteinases.[54] Promising work has been done with types of bone morphogenic protein (BMP), which has been shown to play a role in normal tendon regeneration, and expressed during development to form tendons and their insertion.[58,59] BMP-2 and recombinant human BMP-12 have both been investigated in rotator cuff repair animal models. Both types of BMP have shown promise in providing potential increase in tissue formation and strength between tendon and bone.[60,61] Despite the potential benefit of BMP as an adjuvant, no clinical studies are available as of yet.

Platelet-rich plasma (PRP) is currently used by many surgeons as an augment for rotator cuff repair. PRP is made from taking a sample of a patient's own blood and running it through a centrifuge to leave a high concentration of platelets, which secrete a variety of growth factors thought to be important in healing and angiogenesis.[62]

Clinical studies comparing patients receiving PRP or other similar variants versus a control group who received no additional therapies after rotator cuff repair show no difference in clinical outcomes. These studies also have not shown convincing evidence of improved healing.[63–65]

Biologic and pharmacologic augmentation to enhance rotator cuff repair is still in its infancy. Growth factor augmentation, tissue engineering, stem cells, and gene therapy all have potential roles in therapy. However, the extent of their roles largely depends on being able to fully understand and optimize the biologic environment for rotator cuff tendon healing.[54]

SUMMARY

Rotator cuff disease accounts for more than 4.5 million annual visits to a physician, and more than 75 000 surgical repairs are performed a year.[66] Surgical techniques have evolved from all open repairs to all arthroscopic repairs being the most commonly used. The purpose of this article is to review the current evidence regarding the outcomes of surgical techniques in rotator cuff surgery. Reported outcomes have been favorable with open, mini-open, and arthroscopic repairs. Recently, a committee sponsored by the AAOS published a clinical practice guideline summary regarding the management of rotator cuff tears.[67] The guidelines touched aspects of both nonoperative and operative repair. In regard to operative repair, the committee could not recommend a modality of surgical repair (eg, arthroscopic vs open) as a superior method, citing a lack of comparative studies. The theoretical advantage of arthroscopic surgery lies in smaller soft tissue dissection and the ability to evaluate and treat the glenohumeral joint. However, no study using patient-based outcomes has shown superiority compared with open or mini-open repairs.

With the method of surgical repair not changing outcomes, investigation has recently focused on optimizing bone-tendon healing in rotator cuff repair. Double-row fixation allows for a more anatomic reapproximation of the rotator cuff footprint on the greater tuberosity versus single-row and has been shown to be biomechanically superior. Despite this, no clinical studies have shown superiority of one type of repair versus the other. The AAOS committee citing similar evidence gave a weak recommendation for the use of achieving tendon-to-bone healing with double-row fixation.[67] Transosseous-equivalent repair, which provides a high compressive force on the tendon-to-bone interface of repair, is the newest fixation method under investigation to optimize healing.

The use of collagen and biologic augmentation has gained interest as researchers are attempting to optimize rotator cuff healing. There is moderate evidence against the use of porcine small intestine submucosa xenograft patches.[67] Other commercially available collagen augments have yet to be proven as either beneficial or detrimental. Other than PRP, which has not shown to have any benefit augmenting repair, no biologic augment has been investigated clinically.

Overall, rotator cuff surgery portends a good outcome for appropriately selected patients. However, there is not much high-quality evidence-based research that can be used to conclude what surgical treatments are superior or appropriate for a given patient.[67] Future research should be aimed at identifying whether and in whom rotator cuff healing is appropriate to better identify surgical candidates as well as to determine the best surgical repair strategy.

REFERENCES

1. Bartolozzi A, Andreychik D, Ahmad S. Determinants of outcome in the treatment of rotator cuff disease. Clin Orthop Relat Res 1994;308:90–7.

2. Wolf BR, Dunn WR, Wright RW. Indications for repair of full-thickness rotator cuff tears. Am J Sports Med 2007;35(6):1007–16.
3. Dunn WR, Schackman BR, Walsh C, et al. Variation in orthopaedic surgeons' perceptions about the indications for rotator cuff surgery. J Bone Joint Surg Am 2005;87:1978–84.
4. Favard L, Bacle G, Berhouet J. Rotator cuff repair. Joint Bone Spine 2007;74:551–7.
5. Codmann EA. Complete rupture of the supraspinatus tendon. Operative treatment with report of two successful cases. Boston Med Surg J 1911;164:708–10.
6. Neer CS 2nd. Anterior acromioplasty for the chronic impingement syndrome in the shoulder: a preliminary report. J Bone Joint Surg Am 1972;54:41–50.
7. Bigliani LU, Cordasco FA, McIlveen SJ, et al. Operative treatment of failed repairs of the rotator cuff. J Bone Joint Surg Am 1992;74:1505–15.
8. Ellman H, Hanker G, Bayer M. Repair of the rotator cuff. End-result study of factors influencing reconstruction. J Bone Joint Surg Am 1986;68:1136–44.
9. Gupta R, Leggin BG, Iannotti JP. Results of surgical repair of full-thickness tears of the rotator cuff. Orthop Clin North Am 1997;28:241–8.
10. Rokito AS, Cuomo F, Gallagher MA, et al. Long-term functional outcome of repair of large and massive chronic tears of the rotator cuff. J Bone Joint Surg Am 1999; 81:991–7.
11. Iannotti JP, Bernot MP, Kuhlman JR, et al. Postoperative assessment of shoulder function: a prospective study of full thickness rotator cuff tears. J Shoulder Elbow Surg 1996;5:449–57.
12. Cofield RH, Parvizi J, Hoffmeyer PJ, et al. Surgical repair of chronic rotator cuff tears. A prospective long term study. J Bone Joint Surg Am 2001;83-A:71–7.
13. Hawkins RJ, Misamore GW, Hobeika PE. Surgery for full-thickness rotator-cuff tears. J Bone Joint Surg Am 1985;67:1349–55.
14. Levy HJ, Uribe JW, Delaney LG. Arthroscopic assisted rotator cuff repair: preliminary results. Arthroscopy 1990;6:55–60.
15. Paulos LE, Kody MH. Arthroscopically enhanced "miniapproach" to rotator cuff repair. Am J Sports Med 1994;22:19–25.
16. Liu SH. Arthroscopically assisted rotator-cuff repair. J Bone Joint Surg Br 1994; 76:593–5.
17. Shinners TJ, Noordsij PG, Orwin JF. Arthroscopically assisted mini-open rotator cuff repair. Arthroscopy 2002;18:21–6.
18. Boszotta H, Prunner K. Arthroscopically assisted rotator cuff repair. Arthroscopy 2004;20:620–6.
19. Baker CL, Liu SH. Comparison of open and arthroscopically assisted rotator cuff repairs. Am J Sports Med 1995;1:99–104.
20. Mohtadi NG, Hollinshead RM, Sasyniuk TM, et al. A randomized clinical trial comparing open to arthroscopic acromioplasty with mini-open rotator cuff repair for full-thickness rotator cuff tears: a disease-specific quality of life outcome at an average 2-year follow-up. Am J Sports Med 2008;36:1043–51.
21. Gartsman GM, Khan M, Hammerman SM. Arthroscopic repair of full-thickness tears of the rotator cuff. J Bone Joint Surg Am 1998;80:832–40.
22. Gartsman GM, Hammerman SM. Full-thickness tears: arthroscopic repair. Orthop Clin North Am 1997;28:83–98.
23. Burkhart SS, Danaceau SM, Pearce CE. Arthroscopic rotator cuff repair: analysis of results by tear size and by repair technique-margin convergence versus direct tendon-to-bone repair. Arthroscopy 2001;17:905–12.
24. Burkhart SS, Lo IK. Arthroscopic rotator cuff repair. J Am Acad Orthop Surg 2006; 14:333–46.

25. Morse K, Davis AD, Afra R, et al. Arthroscopic versus mini-open rotator cuff repair: a comprehensive review and meta-analysis. Am J Sports Med 2008;36: 1824–8.
26. Youm T, Murray DH, Kubiak EN, et al. Arthroscopic versus mini-open rotator cuff repair: a comparison of clinical outcomes and patient satisfaction. J Shoulder Elbow Surg 2005;14:455–9.
27. Sauerbrey AM, Getz CL, Piancastelli M, et al. Arthroscopic versus mini-open rotator cuff repair: a comparison of clinical outcome. Arthroscopy 2005;21: 1415–20.
28. Ide J, Maeda S, Takagi K. A comparison of arthroscopic and open rotator cuff repair. Arthroscopy 2005;21:1090–8.
29. Buess E, Steuber KU, Waibl B. Open versus arthroscopic rotator cuff repair: a comparative view of 96 cases. Arthroscopy 2005;21:597–604.
30. Bishop J, Klepps S, Lo IK, et al. Cuff integrity after arthroscopic versus open rotator cuff repair: a prospective study. J Shoulder Elbow Surg 2006;15: 290–9.
31. Galatz LM, Ball CM, Teefey SA, et al. The outcome and repair integrity of completely arthroscopically repaired large and massive rotator cuff tears. J Bone Joint Surg Am 2004;86:219–24.
32. Lichtenberg S, Liem D, Magosch P, et al. Influence of tendon healing after arthroscopic rotator cuff repair on clinical outcome using single-row Mason-Allen suture technique, a prospective MRI controlled study. Knee Surg Sports Traumatol Arthrosc 2006;14:1200–6.
33. Boehm TD, Werner A, Radtke S, et al. The effect of suture material and techniques on the outcome of repair of the rotator cuff: a prospective, randomised study. J Bone Joint Surg Br 2005;87:819–23.
34. Sugaya H, Maeda K, Matsuki K, et al. Functional and structural outcome after arthroscopic full-thickness rotator cuff repair: single-row versus dual-row fixation. Arthroscopy 2005;21:1307–16.
35. Park JY, Lhee SH, Choi JH, et al. Comparison of the clinical outcomes of single- and double-row repairs in rotator cuff tears. Am J Sports Med 2008;36:1310–6.
36. Burks RT, Crim J, Brown N, et al. A prospective randomized clinical trial comparing arthroscopic single- and double-row rotator cuff repair: magnetic resonance imaging and early clinical evaluation. Am J Sports Med 2009;37:674–82.
37. Waltrip RL, Zheng N, Dugas JR, et al. Rotator cuff repair. A biomechanical comparison of three techniques. Am J Sports Med 2003;31:493–7.
38. Meier SW, Meier JD. The effect of double-row fixation on initial repair strength in rotator cuff repair: a biomechanical study. Arthroscopy 2006;22:1168–73.
39. Brady PC, Arrigoni P, Burkhart SS. Evaluation of residual rotator cuff defects after in vivo single- versus double-row rotator cuff repairs. Arthroscopy 2006; 22:1070–5.
40. Wall LB, Keener JD, Brophy RH. Clinical outcomes of double-row versus single-row rotator cuff repairs. Arthroscopy 2009;25:1312–8.
41. Saridakis P, Jones G. Outcomes of single-row and double-row arthroscopic rotator cuff repair: a systematic review. J Bone Joint Surg Am 2010;92:732–42.
42. Franceschi F, Ruzzini L, Longo UG, et al. Equivalent clinical results of arthroscopic single-row and double-row repair for rotator cuff tears: a randomized controlled trial. Am J Sports Med 2007;35:1254–60.
43. Grasso A, Milano G, Salvatore M, et al. Single-row versus double-row arthroscopic rotator cuff repair: a prospective clinical study. Arthroscopy 2009;25:4–12.

44. Burks RT, Crim J, Brown N, et al. A prospective randomized clinical trial comparing arthroscopic single- and double-row rotator cuff repair. Am J Sports Med 2009;37:647–83.
45. Park MC, Elattrache NS, Ahmad CS, et al. "Transosseous-equivalent" rotator cuff repair technique. Arthroscopy 2006;22:1360.e1–5.
46. Park MC, Idjadi JA, Elattrache NS, et al. The effect of dynamic external rotation comparing 2 footprint-restoring rotator cuff repair techniques. Am J Sports Med 2008;36:893–900.
47. Behrens SB, Bruce B, Zonno AJ, et al. Initial fixation strengths of transosseous-equivalent suture bridge rotator cuff repair is comparable with transosseous repair. Am J Sports Med 2012;40:133–40.
48. Toussaint B, Schnaser E, Bosley J, et al. Early structural and functional outcomes for arthroscopic double-row transosseous-equivalent rotator cuff repair. Am J Sports Med 2001;39:1217–25.
49. Ianotti JP, Codsi MJ, Kwon YW, et al. Porcine small intestine submucosa augmentation of surgical repair of chronic two-tendon rotator cuff tears: a randomized controlled trial. J Bone Joint Surg Am 2006;88:1238–44.
50. Schlamber SG, Tibone JE, Itamura JM, et al. Six-month magnetic resonance imaging follow-up of large and massive rotator cuff repairs reinforced with porcine small intestine mucosa. J Shoulder Elbow Surg 2004;13:538–41.
51. Walton JR, Bowman NK, Khatib Y, et al. Restore orthobiologic implant: not recommended for augmentation of rotator cuff repairs. J Bone Joint Surg Am 2007;89:786–91.
52. Badhe SP, Lawrence TM, Smith FD, et al. An assessment of porcine dermal xenograft as an augmentation graft in the treatment of extensive rotator cuff tears. J Shoulder Elbow Surg 2008;17:35–9.
53. Bond JL, Dopirak RM, Higgins J, et al. Arthroscopic replacement of massive, irreparable rotator cuff tears using a GrafJacket allograft: technique and preliminary results. Arthroscopy 2008;24:403–9.
54. Edwards SL, Lynch TS, Saltzman MD, et al. Biologic and pharmacologic augmentation of rotator cuff repairs. J Am Acad Orthop Surg 2011;19:583–9.
55. Carpenter JE, Thomopoulos S, Flanagan CI, et al. Rotator cuff defect healing: a biomechanical and histologic analysis in an animal model. J Shoulder Elbow Surg 1998;7:599–605.
56. Gimbel JA, Van Kleunen JP, Mehta S, et al. Supraspinatus tendon organizational and mechanical properties in a chronic rotator cuff tear animal model. J Biomech 2004;37:739–49.
57. Galatz LM, Sandell LJ, Rothermich SY, et al. Characteristics of the rat supraspinatus tendon during tendon-to-bone healing after acute injury. J Orthop Res 2006;24:541–50.
58. Chuen FS, Chuk CY, Ping WY, et al. Immunohistochemical characterization of cells in adult human patellar tendons. J Histochem Cytochem 2004;52:1151–7.
59. Wofman NM, Hattersley G, Cox K, et al. Ectopic induction of tendon and ligament in rats by growth and differentiation factors of 5, 6, and 7, members of the TGF-beta gene family. J Clin Invest 1997;100:321–30.
60. Rodeo SA, Potter HG, Kawamura S, et al. Biologic augmentation of rotator cuff tendon-healing with use of a mixture of osteoinductive growth factors. J Bone Joint Surg Am 2007;89:2485–97.
61. Seeherman HJ, Archambault JM, Rodeo SA, et al. rhBMP-12 accelerates healing of rotator cuff repairs in a sheep model. J Bone Joint Surg Am 2008;90:2206–19.

62. Creaney L, Hamilton B. Growth factor delivery methods in the management of sports injuries: the state of play. Br J Sports Med 2008;42:314–20.
63. Weber SC, Kauffman JI. Platelet-rich fibrin matrix in arthroscopic rotator cuff repair: a prospective randomized study. Presented at the 77th Annual Meeting of the American Academy of Orthopaedic Surgeons. New Orleans, March 9–13, 2010.
64. Castricini R, Longo UG, De Benedeto M, et al. Platelet-rich plasma augmentation for arthroscopic rotator cuff repair: a randomized controlled trial. Am J Sports Med 2011;39:258–65.
65. Anderson L, Anziano D. Use of platelet rich fibrin matrix in rotator cuff repairs. Presented at the Arthroscopy Association of North America Fall Course. Palm Springs, November 18–20, 2010.
66. Vitale MA, Vitale MG, Zivin JG, et al. Rotator cuff repair: an analysis of utility scores and cost-effectiveness. J Shoulder Elbow Surg 2007;16:181–7.
67. Pedowitz RA, Yamaguchi K, Ahmad CS, et al. Optimizing the management of rotator cuff problems. J Am Acad Orthop Surg 2011;19:368–79.

Rotator Cuff Tears in Overhead Athletes

Kostas J. Economopoulos, MD, Stephen F. Brockmeier, MD*

KEYWORDS

- Rotator cuff tear • Overhead athlete • Internal impingement

KEY POINTS

- Rotator cuff tears in overhead athletes can take on several different forms, including isolated undersurface partial-thickness cuff tears, intratendinous delamination tears (partial articular-sided intrasubstance tear lesion), concomitant partial-thickness tears with labral injury, undersurface partial-thickness tears with capsular injury or insufficiency, partial-thickness bursal-side tears with or without subacromial impingement, or full-thickness rotator cuff tears.
- Identification of symptomatic rotator cuff disease can be challenging in the overhead athlete as abnormalities of the rotator cuff can be seen commonly in asymptomatic throwers and rotator cuff pathologic conditions often occur in conjunction with other injuries.
- Partial-thickness tears treated with arthroscopic debridement and management of concomitant pathologic conditions appear to have fairly good outcomes in the literature with most athletes able to return to activity at their preinjury level. Full-thickness tears, however, have fared much more poorly in the overhead athlete, with largely dismal outcomes after surgical repair.

INTRODUCTION

Although most athletic endeavors can lead to injury of the shoulder and surrounding soft tissues, shoulder injuries in the overhead or throwing athlete can be particularly difficult to manage. Overhead activities impart supraphysiologic stresses on the structures of the shoulder, which can lead to a unique subset of pathologic conditions of the labrum, biceps, and rotator cuff. This has been best studied in baseball pitchers. A tremendous amount of force and torque is generated by the shoulder to create the acceleration necessary for throwing an object at high velocities and decelerating the upper extremity after the ball has been released. A baseball pitch can lead to humeral angular velocities as high as 7000 to 8000°/s and joint compressive loads reaching 860 N.[1,2] Biomechanical studies have clearly identified the muscles of the rotator cuff as the principal dynamic stabilizers that act to offset these high energy

The authors have nothing to disclose.
Department of Orthopaedic Surgery, University of Virginia, 400 Ray C. Hunt Drive, Suite 330, Charlottesville, VA 22908, USA
* Corresponding author.
E-mail address: sfb2e@hscmail.mcc.virginia.edu

forces on the shoulder and stabilize the humeral head within the glenoid. This action leads to tremendous stresses on the rotator cuff, tensile, compressive, and shear, especially during the deceleration phase of throwing.

Rotator cuff tears in overhead athletes can take on several different forms including isolated undersurface partial-thickness cuff tears, intratendinous delamination tears (partial articular-sided intrasubstance tear lesion), concomitant partial-thickness tears with labral injury, undersurface partial-thickness tears with capsular injury or insufficiency, partial-thickness bursal-side tears with or without subacromial impingement, or full-thickness rotator cuff tears.[3] Treatment of each depends on several criteria, such as tear location, the depth or thickness of injury, other associated intra-articular injuries, and patient signs and symptoms. Although conservative management options consisting primarily of rest, physical therapy, and correction of faulty mechanics are clearly the preferred approach in the management of most these injuries, some may fail and require surgical intervention. Although both open and arthroscopic approaches to management of rotator cuff pathologic conditions in this population have been described in the literature, outcomes have been variable and seem to be dependent on the nature and extent of the tear along with associated injuries.

CAUSES

From a mechanical standpoint, rotator cuff tears in athletes have traditionally been attributed to 3 mechanisms: tensile overload, primary impingement, and, most commonly, internal impingement of the shoulder. Primary tensile failure of the rotator cuff refers to partial and intrasubstance rotator cuff failure caused by repeated injury. The rotator cuff muscles are highly active during the pitching motion. The rotator cuff is primarily responsible for generating the glenohumeral compressive load that occurs during throwing. The rotator cuff must not only offset high-energy forces in decelerating the arm after release but also stabilize the humeral head within the glenoid. These eccentric tensile forces can overload the rotator cuff tendons, resulting in microtrauma and failure of the tendon fibers, which can accumulate with repetitive throwing and stress.[4]

Most of the injury is believed to occur during the deceleration phase of throwing. This deceleration requires a rapid and well-coordinated eccentric contraction from the superior and posterior rotator cuff to decelerate the arm from its maximum angular velocity.[5] The eccentric nature of this contraction creates significant stress across the tendons, leading to the potential for tendon injury. If the timing and force of contraction are not adequate, continued rotation of the humerus can result in tensile failure of the rotator cuff fibers.[5] The undersurfaces of the posterior half of the supraspinatus and anterior half of the infraspinatus are most commonly involved. Changes in the vascularity of the rotator cuff associated with aging or other metabolic changes may weaken the tendon and play a role in the pathogenesis of primary tensile failure.[6]

Subacromial impingement has been described as a common etiologic factor in the development of rotator cuff disease in the older population since being described by Neer in 1972.[7] Although less common, overhead athletes may also suffer from subacromial impingement. The acromion, coracoacromial ligament, and coracoid process make up the coracoacromial arch. The soft tissue contents of the subacromial space, including the tendons of the rotator cuff, must pass under the coracoacromial arch for the athlete to elevate the arm at greater than 90°. Overhead actions require maximal abduction with external rotation. This motion subjects the subacromial bursa and rotator cuff tendons to wear below the anterior acromion and coracoacromial ligament as the arm accelerates forward. The bursa is a reactive tissue, and this external mechanical stimulus may initiate a response of intrinsic factors, leading to inflammation and pain.[8–10]

Alternatively, rotator cuff weakness may also lead to impingement caused by mechanical dysfunction and loss of the glenohumeral force coupling mechanism. In this setting, a comparative rotator cuff strength deficit may lead to a loss of counterbalance to the superior pull of the deltoid. The humeral head will migrate superiorly during the throwing motion, which can then lead to rotator cuff outlet impingement.

Poor scapular mechanics may also play a role. Overhead athletes require a fine balance between glenohumeral and scapulothoracic function. The typical scapulothoracic rhythm is a 2:1 ratio of glenohumeral movement to scapulothoracic movement. Altered static and dynamic scapular mechanics may arise from overuse and weakness of scapular stabilizers and posterior rotator cuff muscles.[11] Scapular rotation helps with general range of motion of the shoulder. During cocking, when the humerus is terminally externally rotated and abducted, upward scapular rotation helps maintain glenohumeral articular congruency.[12] Weakness, inflexibility, or imbalance of the periscapular and posterior rotator cuff muscles disturbs the normal anatomic static and dynamic relationships of the scapula and has been termed scapular dyskinesis. Burkhart and colleagues labeled the abnormal motion of the scapula as SICK (scapular malposition, inferior medial border prominence, coracoid pain, and dyskinesis of scapular movement).[13] In this setting, scapular dyskinesis leads the scapula to sit in a protracted and upwardly tilted position, causing the glenoid to face anteriorly and superiorly. Glenoid protraction leads the anterior band of the Inferior Glenohumeral Ligament (IGHL) to tighten, limiting anterior translation of the humeral head and making it susceptible to chronic strain.[14] At the same time, the posterior edge of the glenoid is brought toward the humerus, placing the posterosuperior labrum and rotator cuff at risk for injury. Finally, excessive protraction increases glenohumeral angulation. The arm of a thrower with increased glenohumeral angulation will lag behind the body. The increased external rotation can produce posterosuperior glenoid impingement.[15,16]

In this way, alterations in the scapulohumeral rhythm are potential factors leading to cuff impingement against the coracoacromial arch, culminating in rotator cuff injuries.[5,17,18] Scapular rotation allows the acromion to clear the greater tuberosity as the humerus is elevated. Periscapular muscle weakness may also play an important role in the development of partial rotator cuff tears.[19] A thrower may compensate for a weak serratus anterior by dropping their elbow, which decreases the degree of scapular rotation and elevation needed. If the process continues, the thrower may compensate by moving the humerus behind the scapular plane, worsening hyperabduction. The glenohumeral joint hyperangulates as the elbow falls farther behind the plane of the scapula, resulting in more pronounced impingement.

A commonly identified process in overhead athletes leading to partial articular-sided rotator cuff tears is internal impingement. As originally described by Walch and colleagues,[20–22] internal impingement refers to abnormal contact between the undersurface of the rotator cuff and the superior glenoid and superior labrum that occurs during the throwing motion (**Fig. 1**). During the late cocking and acceleration phases of overhead throwing, forceful and repeated contact of the undersurface of the rotator cuff and the superior labrum can lead to a specific pattern of structural injury, specifically superior labrum anterior posterior lesions and partial-thickness rotator cuff damage, which is characteristically noted in the more posterior aspect of the supraspinatus or the superior aspect of the infraspinatus.[20–23] Burkhart and colleagues[24] proposed posterior capsular contracture as a main factor in the development of internal impingement. They theorized that the posterior capsule must withstand significant tensile forces during the deceleration and follow-through phases of throwing.

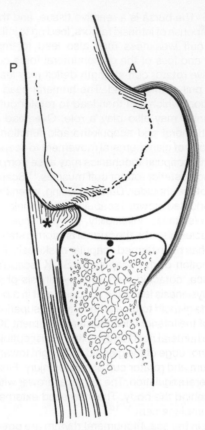

Fig. 1. Internal impingement. As the shoulder becomes fully abducted and externally rotated, the greater tuberosity abuts against the posterosuperior glenoid, entrapping the rotator cuff between the 2 bones. The impinged rotator cuff is represented by the *asterisk*. A, anterior; C, glenohumeral center of rotation; P, posterior. (*From* Burkhart SS, Morgan CD, Kibler WB. The disabled throwing shoulder: spectrum of pathology, part I: pathoanatomy and biomechanics. Arthroscopy 2003;19:406; with permission.)

Eccentric contraction of the rotator cuff, mainly the infraspinatus and posterior capsule, is the primary restraint to these posterior tensile forces. Repeated contraction of the infraspinatus and posterior capsule can cause hypertrophy and stiffness of these structures. Eventually, the infraspinatus and posterior capsule become contracted. This contracture shifts the center of rotation of the shoulder to a more posterosuperior location, leading to posterosuperior instability with the shoulder in abduction and external rotation. The cumulative effect of this cascade of events allows the humeral head to externally hyperrotate, producing increased shear in the rotator cuff tendon and more pronounced internal impingement.

Although there are 3 primary mechanisms that can cause rotator cuff tears in overhead athletes, a component of each may come into play with these tears. Seldom does one single event lead to a rotator cuff injury in the overhead athlete population. By identifying the pathologic factors that lead to rotator cuff injury early, we may be able to prevent further progression and possibly avoid season or career ending surgery.

EVALUATION OF ROTATOR CUFF TEARS IN OVERHEAD ATHLETES
History

Because most overhead athletes with rotator cuff tears do not present with a single, isolated traumatic event, the history is more commonly a gradual onset of pain that progressively becomes worse with increased overhead sports activity.[25] Typical chief complaints are shoulder pain and decreased pitch velocity. A careful history describing the details of any specific aggravating event or precipitation of symptoms is useful in making the diagnosis. Rotator cuff–based pain is typically referred laterally and radiates to the region of the deltoid. Anterior shoulder pain in the region of the joint line can be seen with a superior labral or proximal biceps pathologic condition. Anterior shoulder pain around the coracoid may also be a sign of anterior capsulolabral injury. Posterior joint line pain can be associated with a posterior labral pathologic condition. Pain precipitators and duration should be elucidated: Is the pain associated only with overhead sports, or does the patient have baseline pain or even nocturnal symptoms that awakens him or her from sleep? Concomitant symptoms of instability should also be documented. These may include a feeling of the arm going "dead" or the sensation of subluxation. Pitchers with anterior instability will typically experience the greatest discomfort during the late cocking or early acceleration phase. Pitchers with posterior instability, on the other hand, will complain of pain during the follow-phase of throwing.

Physical Examination

As with all shoulder injuries, a comprehensive physical examination is critical. Specific attention must be given to rotator cuff strength testing, shoulder stability, capsular laxity, and scapular rotation with shoulder motion. Rotator cuff strength in athletes with tears can be altered as a result of pain, poor mechanics, tendon deficit, or, in the unusual circumstance, suprascapular neuropathy. Assessment of each musculotendinous unit of the rotator cuff should be performed using the contralateral arm as a comparison; impingement tests (ie, Neer and Hawkins tests) should also be performed. During examination, it is key to determine whether any positive test truly recreates the athlete's presenting pain or symptoms.

Range of motion of the shoulder should also be closely evaluated. Loss of internal rotation while the arm is abducted to 90° indicates a contracture of the posterior aspect of the shoulder. Contracture of the posterior capsule may lead to increased stress on the anterior labrum and capsule, possibly with subsequent laxity. The glenohumeral capsule and labrum maintain the stability of the glenohumeral joint. Ligamentous stability is tested in the anterior, posterior, and inferior directions and is mandatory in the young athlete because of the possibility of a coexistent internal impingement.[26] Laxity of these structures can be determined by identifying increased translation of the glenohumeral joint in addition to an increase in passive rotation compared with the opposite shoulder.

The examiner must also differentiate between normal thrower's laxity and pathologic laxity. The focus should be on whether the athlete's symptoms are recreated with translation of the joint. The shoulder should be tested for anterior, posterior, and inferior laxity with the arm adducted and with the arm abducted to 90°.[9,27] Signs of labral injury should be sought. The relocation maneuver reproduces the maximal-cocking phase of the throw.[28] If a posterior labral lesion or a posterior lesion of internal impingent is present, this maneuver reproduces posterior joint line pain. The active compression maneuver of O'Brien reproduces anterior joint line pain if an anterosuperior or internal impingement is present.[25,29]

Scapular rotation is evaluated by having the patient elevate the arms overhead and comparing the scapular mechanics between the symptomatic and asymptomatic arms. Asymmetry between the 2 sides is consistent with scapular dyskinesis. Scapular winging, when present, must be identified. Neurologic scapular winging is uncommon; however, long thoracic neuropathy represents a potentially reversible cause of secondary rotator cuff impingement and should not be missed.[5] If long thoracic neuropathy is suspected on physical examination, it should be confirmed with electromyography.[30] Poor scapular mechanics may contribute considerably to rotator cuff–related symptoms and must be corrected to return the athlete to competition.[25]

Another potential cause of anterior impingement–like pain is suprascapular neuropathy. The most common physical finding with chronic suprascapular neuropathy is supraspinatus and infraspinatus atrophy. In the young, athletic population, rotator cuff tears large enough to cause atrophy of the supraspinatus and infraspinatus are uncommon. Therefore, these findings in the young overhead athlete are more consistent with suprascapular neuropathy.[31] If suprascapular neuropathy is suspected, further testing should be performed (electromyography).

Imaging

Plain radiographs, although routinely obtained, are frequently unremarkable. Although nonspecific, enthesopathic changes at the greater tuberosity, including notching and cystic changes, have been associated with partial-thickness articular-surface tears in throwing athletes.[32] Axillary and anteroposterior views of the shoulder should be reviewed for abnormal calcifications. The acromial shape is evaluated with an outlet view to determine if outlet impingement is present. Other potentially helpful views include anteroposterior views in internal and external rotation and a West Point view.

Magnetic resonance imaging (MRI) is the imaging modality of choice in the evaluation of athletes with a suspected rotator cuff pathologic condition. Smith and colleagues[33] performed a meta-analysis looking at the accuracy of MRI in detecting partial and complete rotator cuff tears. The study found that for partial-thickness rotator cuff tears, the pooled sensitivity and specificity were 0.80 and 0.95, respectively. For full-thickness tears, the sensitivity and specificity values were 0.91 and 0.97, respectively. Factors that lead to improved accuracy were images read by musculoskeletal radiologists and higher-field strength (3.0 T) MRI. Other studies evaluating the use of standard MRI have shown only moderate success in diagnosing partial-thickness tears. Sensitivity rates between 56% and 72% and specificity rates of 85% for tears confirmed with arthroscopy have been described.[34] Gartsman and Milne reported a false-negative rate of 83% when they evaluated 12 arthroscopically verified articular-sided partial thickness tears.[35]

Image enhancement with use intra-articular contrast or specialized sequences can improve accuracy in identifying rotator cuff tears (**Fig. 2**). Magnetic resonance arthrography with coronal oblique fat-suppression sequences has a reported sensitivity of 84% and a specificity of 96% with an overall accuracy of 91% in identifying partial-cuff tears.[36] Lee and Lee demonstrated that placing the arm in throwing position with the arm abducted and externally rotated improves the detection of rotator cuff tears.[37] The sensitivity for detecting articular and intratendinous rotator cuff tears using standard magnetic resonance arthrography in the coronal oblique view was 21%. The sensitivity increased to 100% using the arm abducted and externally rotated sequence.

Ultrasound has also been shown to be an effective tool in diagnosing both partial- and full-thickness rotator cuff tears. A recent meta-analysis showed a sensitivity and

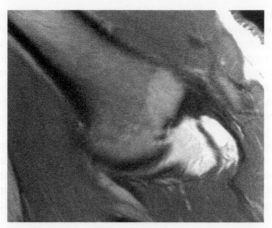

Fig. 2. Coronal image of a partial rotator cuff tear with the arm in the abducted externally rotator position. Significant intrasubstance delamination of the tissue is seen in addition to a partial rotator cuff tear.

specificity of 0.84 and 0.89, respectively, for partial-thickness tears and 0.96 and 0.93, respectively, for full-thickness rotator cuff tears using ultrasound.[38] Wiener and Seitz reported a sensitivity of 94% and specificity of 93% for the diagnosis of partial-thickness rotator cuff tears using ultrasound.[39] Although there are several benefits to the use of ultrasound in the diagnosis of rotator cuff tears in athletes, including its ability to dynamically assess the cuff, patient tolerance, and cost, it is highly operator dependent.[40] Because of this key limitation, ultrasound remains primarily used only in certain centers, and magnetic resonance arthrography remains the more commonly used imaging modality in this clinical scenario.

TREATMENT OPTIONS IN THE OVERHEAD ATHLETE WITH A ROTATOR CUFF PATHOLOGIC CONDITION

Several factors are taken into account when determining the best approach to the management of rotator cuff tears in overhead athletes; treatment is determined by the specific nature of the injury and tailored for each patient and situation. A few of the factors that must be considered when planning the treatment of these patients are whether the tear is partial or full thickness, whether it is caused by internal or external forces, the extent of the athlete's degree of impairment, whether it is an in-season or out-of-season injury, and other associated pathologic conditions. In almost every case, an initial attempt at nonsurgical management is favored. Athletes with minor injuries typically respond to rest within 3 months and are able to return to throwing.[1] If nonoperative treatment fails, then surgical intervention is necessary.

Nonoperative Treatment

Rest and activity modification in addition to nonsteroidal anti-inflammatory drugs are the primary treatment modalities used in nonoperative treatment in overhead athletes with rotator cuff tears. An evaluation of the athlete's throwing mechanics is also critical to potentially identify causative mechanical factors or flaws. In certain situations, subacromial and intra-articular injections may also be used in these patients to decrease inflammation and assist in the rehabilitation and recovery process.

In the overhead athlete, shoulder rehabilitation should focus on maximizing range of motion and strengthening the rotator cuff and periscapular musculature.[40] Anterior and posterior capsular tightness is dealt with using specific stretching exercises. Posterior capsular contracture (glenohumeral internal rotation deficit) is one of the more common causes for shoulder pain in the overhead athlete and is frequently seen in association with rotator cuff disease in this population. When this is present, focused stretches of the posterior capsule can be very helpful in improving joint motion and diminishing shoulder; this is best accomplished using sleeper stretches (**Fig. 3**).

Scapular dyskinesis is approached by restoring the proper scapular-thoracic mechanics using a progressive strengthening program. The scapular muscle activity is integrated by having the athlete retract the scapula into its normal anatomic position. Emphasis on scapulothoracic muscle function during all rotator cuff and deltoid strengthening exercise facilitates scapular muscle integration into sports-specific activities.[5]

Operative Treatment

It should be emphasized that, with only a few notable exceptions, conservative options should be exhausted in this patient population before consideration of surgical intervention. In general, the indications for surgery in an overhead athlete with a rotator cuff tear are the same as those in nonathletes. However, given what is known about the outcomes of rotator cuff surgery in this particularly challenging group of patients, in most cases it is prudent to forego consideration for surgery for a reasonable period ($\geq$3 months) and proceed only after it is clear that the athlete's symptoms are not responding to the available nonsurgical options and it has been demonstrated clearly that a return to play is not feasible.

Once the determination has been made that surgical intervention is warranted, these injuries are generally treated in a similar fashion to that for a conventional rotator cuff pathologic condition. Timing of surgery can depend on whether the athlete is in or out of season. An athlete who is in-season may attempt to treat or manage his or her rotator cuff injury conservatively to get through the season before proceeding to surgery.

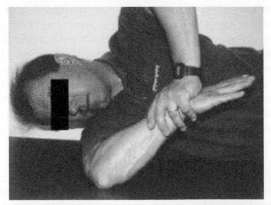

Fig. 3. In the sleep stretch, the patient lies on the side and stabilizes the scapula against the wall. Both the shoulder and the elbow are flexed 90°. The nonaffected arm applies internal rotation to the affected arm. (*From* Burkhart SS, Morgan CD, Kibler WB. The disabled throwing shoulder: spectrum of pathology part I: pathoanatomy and biomechanics. Arthroscopy 2003;19:408; with permission.)

Full-thickness Tears

Full-thickness tears of the rotator cuff in the overhead athlete population are approached much like those in the nonathletic population. Restoring the rotator cuff tendon to its anatomic position on the footprint is the goal of surgical intervention, in addition to optimizing the healing environment of the repair site. This is accomplished by maximizing the contact area between the healing tendon and the bony footprint. A linked, double-row footprint-restoring repair approach (suture-bridge repair or "transosseous-equivalent" technique) offers several potential biomechanical advantages compared with single-row repair and has become increasingly favored (**Fig. 4**). This technique decreases the amount of gap formation, which improves the biomechanical strength of the repair.[41] Additionally, the suture-bridge construct does not rely as much on the lateral tendon tissue to hold suture. This lateral tissue is commonly the more compromised portion of the tendon after a rotator cuff tear.

A key to successful repair of a full-thickness rotator cuff tear in overhead athletes is avoiding overtensioning the repair. Sutures passed too far medially will overtighten the repair, possibly leading to excessive strain and likely failure.[42] The medial row is placed on the lateral edge of the normal bare area on the humeral head if the posterior supraspinatus and infraspinatus are involved.[43,44] This is a crucial concept to keep in mind, as this area of the tendon insertion is more commonly affected in this population. Any alteration of the normal anatomy of the rotator cuff insertion by medializing the repair into the bare area will theoretically alter the mechanics of shoulder motion and likely lead to diminished outcomes in the overhead athlete population.

Partial-thickness Tears

The treatment of partial-thickness rotator cuff tears depends on several factors, including the depth of the tear, location of the tear, quality of the tissue, and the patient's age, sport, and position. Surgical options include debridement of the rotator cuff tear, tear completion and subsequent full-thickness repair, transtendinous repair, and intratendinous repair constructs. The decision to debride or repair a rotator cuff tear is primarily made by determining the percentage of tendon thickness that has been compromised. In the general population, the conventional rule of thumb is a tear of less than 50% is debrided, whereas tears of 50% or greater are more suitable for repair. These guidelines have been adopted by several authors for overhead

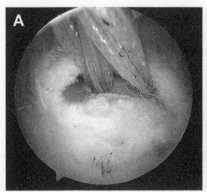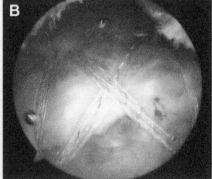

Fig. 4. (*A*) Crescent-shaped full-thickness tear of the supraspinatus with 2 double-loaded anchors placed at the articular margin. (*B*) Suture-bridge repair of the full-thickness tear. Two medial and 2 lateral anchors were used for the repair.

athletes.[1,45,46] However, recently, Rudzki and Shaffer[40] contended that partial tears in the overhead population may be different than those in the nonthrowing patient. They emphasize the high forces endured by the rotator cuff and exaggerated positions the arm must be placed in after surgery, which may threaten the repair in this subset of patients. Because of this, the authors advocate that a partial tear should approach 75% or greater to be considered for repair in overhead athletes.

Articular-sided partial rotator cuff tears that do not meet the criteria for repair are debrided down to healthy, stable tissue using an arthroscopic shaver. When an articular-sided partial tear of 50% to 75% is identified on diagnostic arthroscopy, surgical repair is favored. One option for repair of rotator cuff tears in these patients is to complete the tear and repair it with suture anchors. However, Lo and Burkhart pointed out that after the soft tissue is debrided and brought over laterally to the footprint, a length–tension mismatch of the repaired rotator cuff muscle may occur.[45] Because of these concerns, this group described a transtendinous approach to articular-sided partial rotator cuff tears greater than 50% of the tendon thickness. The technique restores the medial aspect of the footprint while maintaining the lateral footprint of the rotator cuff. This procedure potentially minimizes the length–tendon mismatch.

The technique of transtendon repair is as follows. After routine diagnostic arthroscopy, the partial articular-sided tear is evaluated from within the glenohumeral joint and debrided to a stable margin.[45] Tears making up greater than 6 mm of the footprint are repaired. A non-braided suture is placed through the tear so that the tear may be accurately evaluated on the bursal side. Before repairing the tendon, a complete bursectomy and acromioplasty is performed for better visualization. Evaluation of the tissue marked by the non-braided suture is performed to confirm the tear is truly partial thickness and does not have substantial bursal-side involvement. If the intact bursal tissue is of poor quality, then completion of the tear is favored and the tear repaired with suture anchors. However, if the tissue is reasonable for transtendinous repair, the arthroscope is reintroduced into the glenohumeral joint. An 18-guage spinal needle is placed just lateral to the acromion and directed at the medial margin of the rotator footprint at a 45° angle. A punch is introduced percutaneously through a small stab wound. The punch penetrates the rotator cuff parallel with the 18-gauge needle and creates an anchor socket at the medial margin of the rotator cuff footprint. A suture anchor is then placed percutaneously through the tendon into the socket. If the defect is large enough, a second anchor is placed in the same manner 1 cm posterior to the first anchor. The arthroscope is then reintroduced into the subacromial space and the limbs of the suture anchor are identified. For a 2-anchor repair, 1 limb from each anchor is grasped and brought out through the lateral portal. These sutures are tied together over an instrument. The opposite ends of the suture are pulled leading the tied knot to be drawn into the subacromial space through the cannula and over the top of the rotator cuff. Tension is placed on the 2 untied limbs as they are brought out through the lateral portal and a nonsliding knot is tied. A bridge of suture over the rotator cuff is created that compresses the tendon down to its footprint. If a single-suture anchor is used, a suture passer is used to pass 1 limb of each suture through a more posterior area of the tendon, creating a tissue bridge. The sutures are then tied arthroscopically in the subacromial space, compressing the tendon down over its footprint.

Partial articular-sided tears of the posterior supraspinatus and anterior infraspinatus with a significant intratendinous delamination component can be treated using an intratendinous repair as originally described by Conway (**Fig. 5**).[46,47] A comprehensive diagnostic arthroscopy of the glenohumeral joint is performed with special attention

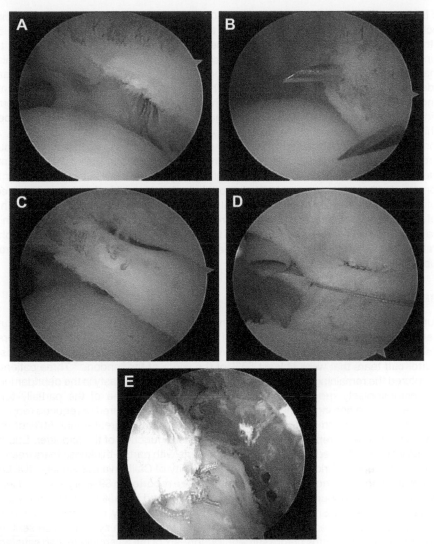

Fig. 5. Intratendinous repair of a partial articular sided tear. (*A*) Intra-articular view of a partial articular sided tear involving the posterior aspect of the supraspinatus and anterior infraspinatus with intratendinous delamination. (*B*) The partial-thickness is held reduced while 2 percutaneous spinal needles\ are placed through the rotator cuff tendon. (*C*) A non-braided suture is passed down each needle and bought through the anterior portal. The sutures are tied together and the knot is shuttled externally. (*D*) A number 2 nonabsorbable suture is then shuttled through the tendon, replacing the previously placed non-braided suture. (*E*) The sutures are retrieved in the subacromial space and tied arthroscopically, creating a mattress suture, reducing the articular-sided partial defect, and closing down the intrasubstance delamination.

placed on the posterosuperior glenoid and labrum to identify concurrent pathologic conditions. The next step is evaluation of the articular side of the rotator cuff. The authors recommend examining the cuff from anterior to posterior with the extremity in 45° of abduction and external rotation to better visualize the more posterior aspect of the supraspinatus and infraspinatus; a 70° arthroscope may also be useful for this technique. An arthroscopic shaver is used to debride the tear including the region of intratendinous extension and to prepare the exposed area of rotator cuff footprint to stimulate a healing response. The arthroscope is redirected into the subacromial space and a complete bursectomy is performed to improve visualization. The bursal side of the area is evaluated to confirm the absence of bursal-sided involvement. Once the bursectomy is complete, the arthroscope is returned to the glenohumeral joint. The partial-thickness flap is held in the reduced position using a tissue grasper while 2 percutaneous spinal needles are placed through the rotator cuff tendon. A non-braided suture is passed down each spinal needle, grasped, and brought out through the anterior portal. The sutures are tied together and pulled into the joint. The knot is then shuttled externally by pulling on 1 end of the suture. A number 2 nonabsorbable suture is then shuttled through the tendon, replacing the non-braided suture. This process can be repeated until the entire tear has been closed down. The sutures are then retrieved from the subacromial space and arthroscopically tied. This creates a mattress construct that fixes the torn articular-sided flap to the intact peripheral rotator cuff, reducing the articular-side partial defect, and closing down the intrasubstance delamination.

TREATMENT OUTCOMES

Outcomes following debridement for the management of partial-thickness rotator cuff tears have varied in the literature. Much of the literature has focused on nonthrowers. Weber compared surgical debridement with mini-open repair of partial-thickness rotator cuff tears that were at least 50% of the width of the tendon.[48] Three patients reruptured the remaining cuff later despite adequate acromioplasty in the debridement and acromioplasty group. At second-look arthroscopy, none of the partially torn tendons showed healing. In the repair group, no patient reruptured or required reoperation. The group recommended that significant partial tears greater than 50% of the tendon thickness be repaired for improved long-term function of the shoulder. Budoff and colleagues[49] looked at 79 shoulders in patients with partial-thickness tears treated with arthroscopic debridement. Using the University of California Los Angeles (UCLA) shoulder rating scale, good to excellent results were reported in 89% of patients at less than 5 years of follow-up. However, this number dropped to 81% when follow-up was longer than 5 years. Snyder and colleagues[50] retrospectively reviewed 31 patients treated with debridement of their partial rotator cuff repair with symptoms present for an average of 20.5 months before surgery. Twenty-six of the 31 shoulders had satisfactory results, whereas the other 5 had unsatisfactory results. The results with and without subacromial decompression were similar. Cordasco and colleagues[51] reviewed 162 with normal, frayed, or partial-thickness rotator cuff tears. Patients with partial-thickness bursal-sided rotator cuff tears (grade 2B) had a significantly higher failure rate (38%). Although the clinical outcome of patients with partial-thickness tears of the rotator cuff consisting of less than 50% of the tendon (grades 1 and 2) was not significantly different from that of patients without partial rotator cuff tears, the subgroup of patients with grade 2B partial tears had a statistically significantly higher failure rate. The authors concluded this subgroup may have been better served with primary repair. No progress of symptoms was identified with 10-year follow-up in patients with partial-thickness tears treated with arthroscopic acromioplasty.

Looking more specifically at throwers, Payne and colleagues[52] evaluated 43 athletes younger than 40 years with partial rotator cuff tears treated with arthroscopic debridement and subacromial decompression at an average of 2-year follow-up.

Three-quarters of the patients were overhead athletes. Payne and colleagues broke up the cohort into those with acute onset and those with insidious onset of pain. Of 14 patients with acute, traumatic injuries, 12 (86%) had satisfactory postoperative results, with 9 returning to preinjury sport. The other group consisted of 29 overhead athletes with insidious, atraumatic shoulder pain. Of these 29 patients, 19 (66%) had satisfactory results and 13 (45%) returned to preinjury sports. Andrews and colleagues[53] reported their results of 36 patients with partial tears of the supraspinatus who underwent arthroscopic debridement of the lesion. All patients were competitive athletes, with 64% being a baseball pitcher. Of 34 patients available for follow-up, 26 (76%) had excellent results, 3 (9%) had good results, and 5 (15%) had poor results. Eighty-five percent of the patients were able to return to their preoperative level of play. They concluded that surgical debridement of partial-thickness rotator cuff tears initiated a healing response. Reynolds and colleagues[54] reported on 82 professional pitchers with small partial-thickness rotator cuff tears treated with debridement. Seventy-six percent of the throwers were able to return to competitive pitching at the professional level, whereas 55% were able to return to the same or higher level of competition. The group concluded that debridement alone of small partial-thickness tears was an effective treatment and allowed the pitchers to return to competition at a similar or higher level in most of the patients.

Partial-thickness tears consisting of 50% or greater of the rotator cuff thickness are typically repaired in both the general population and overhead athletes. It should be noted that 50% seems to be an arbitrary number, and there are no studies establishing this number, especially in this specific population of overhead athletes. Improvement in arthroscopic techniques, poor outcomes with debridement alone, and the concern for progression of partial tears greater than 50% the tendon thickness have led many to repair these tears more frequently.[40] Most bursal-sided partial-thickness tears greater than 50% are treated with completion of the tear and standard repair using suture anchors. Wright and Cofield evaluated their results with partial-thickness tears.[55] They treated 39 patients with open acromioplasty, debridement of abnormal tissue, and tendon suturing. During a 55-month follow-up period, 59% of patients had excellent results, 26% had satisfactory results, and 15% had unsatisfactory results. They concluded that treatment of partial-thickness tears with open acromioplasty, debridement, and tendon repair is effective. Deutsch looked at 41 patients with partial-thickness tears of greater than 50% thickness that were converted to full-thickness tears and repaired with suture anchors.[56] None of the patients were overhead athletes. During a follow-up period of 38 months, all patients had improvement in range of motion and strength. Significant improvement was seen in the American Shoulder and Elbow Surgeons scores and pain relief. The study showed successful results with completion of partial-thickness tears greater than 50% and repair with suture anchors in nonoverhead athletes.

A recent study by Shin compared the repair of symptomatic partial-thickness artic-ular-sided tears greater than 50% using a transtendon repair technique or tear completion and anchor repair.[57] The study evaluated 24 patients randomized to each technique 6 months after surgery. Both groups showed significant improvement with 22 of 24 patients in each group reporting satisfaction with the surgery. However, shoulder function and range of shoulder motion recovered in the patients treated with completion of the tear and anchor repair. Patients in the transtendon group had significantly more pain until 3 months after surgery. MRI performed on all shoulders at 6 months showed all patients in the transtendon group achieved complete integrity, whereas 2 of the 24 patients in the completion and anchor group had retears. In their initial description of the transtendon approach, Lo and Burkhart described their 1-year follow-up.[45] Of the 25 patients in the study, none were overhead athletes. The group described significant improvement in all patients with mean UCLA shoulder scores increasing from a preoperative value of 15 to a postoperative value of 32. Ide and colleagues[58] reported their results of transtendon repair of partial-thickness articular sided tears of the rotator cuff. The study evaluated 17 patients with a mean follow-up of 39 months. The mean UCLA and Japanese Orthopedic Association scores increased significantly from 17.3 and 68.4 points to 32.9 and 94.8 points, respectively, postoperatively. Six patients were overhead throwers with 2 returning to their previous level, 3 returning to a lower level, and 1 patient unable to return to throwing. Waibl and Buess[59] described their results of 22 patients undergoing transtendon repair of a partial articular surface tendon avulsion lesion. None of the patients were athletes. They reported improvement in the UCLA score from a preoperative value of 17.1 to a postoperative value of 31.2 ($P<.01$). Twenty of the 22 patients were satisfied with their results. Excellent or good results were reported in 19 (86%) of 22 patients, 2 patients had fair results, and 1 patient had a poor outcome.

Conway described his initial experience in treating the delaminated intratendinous partial-thickness tear (partial articular-sided intrasubstance tear lesion) using an intra-tendinous repair in overhead athletes.[47] A group of 14 baseball players were followed, including 13 pitchers and 1 outfielder, for an average of 16 months. All the athletes had associated superior labrum anterior posterior tears, whereas 50% had anterior instability. Eight (89%) of 9 patients followed for longer than 1 year were able to return to play at the same or higher level. The 1 player who did not return to his previous level was able to pitch pain-free but could not recover his velocity. Brockmeier and colleagues[46] looked at their short-term results of intratendinous repair of partial-thickness tears in overhead athletes. Eight overhead athletes with a mean follow-up of 5 months showed encouraging initial outcomes. The initial results of transtendon and intratendinous repair of partial rotator cuff tears in overhead athletes look promising, but further study is required to evaluate this technique efficacy.

In general, surgical repair of full-thickness tears in overhead athletes has shown less than ideal results. Tibone and colleagues[60] reviewed 45 athletes with partial or complete rotator cuff tears. All the patients were treated with open anterior acromioplasty and repair of the tear. Fifteen of the athletes had a complete tear of the rotator cuff. Twelve of the 29 athletes who were overhead athletes were able to return to their preinjury level of competition. However, of 5 professional pitchers with full-thickness tears, 3 were unable to return to professional baseball. Two of the 5 were able to return to professional pitching but with significant difficulty. Mazoue and Andrews reported their results in treating 16 professional baseball players with full-thickness rotator cuff tears using a mini-open approach.[61] They looked at 12 pitchers and 4 position players with a mean follow-up of 66 months. The results were poor, with only 1 of the 12 pitchers able to return to his preinjury level. One of 2 positional players with repair of their dominant arm was able to return to his previous level, and both positional players with repair of their nondominant arm were able to return to their preinjury level of play. The authors concluded that return to pitching at the professional level is difficult after repair of a full-thickness rotator cuff tear repaired with a mini-open approach.

SUMMARY

The rotator cuff is under significant stress during overhead athletics, which can predictably lead to a certain spectrum of rotator cuff injuries in this population. Although the cause is often multifactorial; tensile overload, outlet impingement, and internal impingement are common causes of cuff pathologic conditions in this group.

Identification of symptomatic rotator cuff disease can be challenging in the overhead athlete because abnormalities of the rotator cuff are common in asymptomatic throwers and rotator cuff pathologic conditions often occur in conjunction with other injuries. Although nonoperative options should be exhausted, surgical treatment is typically necessary for any rotator cuff tear for which conservative treatment fails. Tear thickness has been classically used to determine the surgical approach, with tears involving less than 50% of the tendon thickness treated with debridement and more substantial tears treated with formal repair. However, some authors and some noted surgeons with experience in managing this patient population have more recently advocated a higher threshold of tendon involvement before considering formal repair.

Multiple repair options have been described, but few reports have focused specifically on the outcomes of rotator cuff surgery in overhead athletes. The limited available data do lead, however, to a few reasonable conclusions. Surgical results typically correlate with tear severity. Partial-thickness tears treated with arthroscopic debridement and management of concomitant pathologic conditions seem to have fairly good outcomes in the literature, with most athletes able to return to activity at their preinjury level. Full-thickness tears, however, have fared much more poorly in the overhead athlete, with largely dismal outcomes after surgical repair. What is abundantly clear is that further refinement of surgical options is necessary to improve patient outcomes after rotator cuff repair in this particularly challenging patient population and to allow more consistent return to sports.

REFERENCES

1. Dillman CJ, Fleisig GS, Andrews JR. Biomechanics of pitching with emphasis upon shoulder kinematics. J Orthop Sports Phys Ther 1993;18:402–8.
2. Gainor BJ, Piotrowski G, Puhl J, et al. The throw: biomechanics and acute injury. Am J Sports Med 1980;8:114–8.
3. Altchek DW, Hatch JD. Rotator cuff injuries in overhead athletes. Oper Tech Orthop 2001;11(1):2–8.
4. Park SS, Loebenberg MI, Rokito AS, et al. The shoulder in baseball pitching: biomechanics and related injuries: part 2. Bull Hosp Jt Dis 2002–2003;61:80–8.
5. Williams GR, Kelley M. Management of rotator cuff and impingement injuries in the athlete. J Athl Train 2000;35(3):300–15.
6. Fakuda H. The management of partial-thickness tears of the rotator cuff. J Bone Joint Surg Br 2003;85:3–11.
7. Neer CS II. Anterior acromioplasty for the chronic impingement syndrome in the shoulder: a preliminary report. J Bone Joint Surg Am 1972;54:41–50.
8. Cofield RH, Simonet WT. The shoulder in sports. Mayo Clin Proc 1984;59:157–64.
9. Hawkins RJ, Kennedy JC. Impingement syndrome in athletes. Am J Sports Med 1980;8:151–8.
10. Jackson DW. Chronic rotator cuff impingement in the throwing athlete. Am J Sports Med 1976;4:231–40.
11. Burkhart SS, Morgan CD, Kibler WB. The disabled throwing shoulder: spectrum of pathology, part II: evaluation and treatment of SLAP lesions in throwers. Arthroscopy 2003;19(5):531–9.
12. Myers JB, Laudner KG, Pasquale MR, et al. Scapular position and orientation in throwing athletes. Am J Sports Med 2005;33(2):263–71.
13. Burkhart SS, Morgan CD, Kibler WB. The disabled throwing shoulder: spectrum of pathology part III: the SICK scapula, scapular dyskinesis, the kinetic chain and rehabilitation. Arthroscopy 2003;19(6):641–61.

14. Weiser WM, Lee TQ, McMaster WC, et al. Effects of simulated scapular protraction on anterior glenohumeral stability. Am J Sports Med 1999;27(6):801–5.
15. Kibler WB. The role of the scapula in athletic shoulder function. Am J Sports Med 1998;26(2):325–37.
16. Kibler WB, McMullen J. Scapular dyskinesis and its relation to shoulder pain. J Am Acad Orthop Surg 2003;11(2):142–51.
17. Warner JP, Micheli LJ, Arslanian LE, et al. Patterns of flexibility, laxity, and strength in normal shoulders and shoulders with instability and impingement. Am J Sports Med 1990;18:366–75.
18. Hawkins RJ, Janda DH, Mohtadi H. The athlete's shoulder. Perspect Orthop Surg 1990;1:1–27.
19. Glousman R, Jobe F, Tibone J, et al. Dynamic electromyography analysis of the throwing shoulder with glenohumeral instability. J Bone Joint Surg Am 1988;70(2):220–6.
20. Walch G, Boileau J, Noel E, et al. Impingement of the deep surface of the supraspinatus tendon on the posterosuperior glenoid rim: an arthroscopic study. J Shoulder Elbow Surg 1992;1:238–43.
21. Jobe CM. Posterior superior glenoid impingement: expanded spectrum. Arthroscopy 1995;11:530–6.
22. Welch G, Liotard JP, Boileau P, et al. Postero-superior glenoid impingement. Another impingement of the shoulder. J Radiol 1993;74:47–50.
23. Jobe CM. Superior glenoid impingement. Orthop Clin North Am 1997;28(2):137–43.
24. Burkhart SS, Morgan CD, Kibler WB. The disabled throwing shoulder: spectrum of pathology part I: pathoanatomy and biomechanics. Arthroscopy 2003;19(4):404–20.
25. Kvitne RS, Jobe FW. The diagnosis and treatment of anterior instability in the throwing athlete. Clin Orthop 1993;291:107–23.
26. Matava MJ, Purcell DB, Rudzki JR. Partial-thickness rotator cuff tear. Am J Sports Med 2005;33:1405–7.
27. Ticker JB, Fealy S, Fu FH. Instability and impingement in the athlete's shoulder. Sports Med 1995;19:418–26.
28. Jobe FW. Impingement problems in the athlete. Instr Course Lect 1989;38:205–9.
29. Miniaci A, Fowler PJ. Impingement in the athlete. Clin Sports Med 1993;12:91–110.
30. Gregg JR, Labosky D, Harty M, et al. Serratus anterior paralysis in the young athlete. J Bone Joint Surg Am 1979;61:825–32.
31. Williams G. Painful shoulder after surgery for rotator cuff disease. J Am Acad Orthop Surg 1997;5:97–108.
32. Nakagawa S, Yoneda M, Hayashida K, et al. Greater tuberosity notch: an important indicator of articular-side partial rotator cuff tears in the shoulders of throwing athletes. Am J Sports Med 2001;29:762–70.
33. Smith TO, Daniell H, Geere JA, et al. The diagnostic accuracy of MRI for the detection of partial- and full-thickness rotator cuff tears in adults. Magn Reson Imaging 2012;30:336–46.
34. Traughber PD, Goodwin TE, Shoulder MR. Arthroscopic correlation with emphasis on partial tears. J Comput Assist Tomogr 1992;16:129–33.
35. Gartsman GM, Milne JC. Articular surface partial-thickness rotator cuff tears. J Shoulder Elbow Surg 1995;4:409–15.
36. Meister K, Thesing J, Montgomery WJ, et al. MR arthrography of partial thickness tears of the undersurface of the rotator cuff: an arthroscopic correlation. Skeletal Radiol 2004;33:136–41.

37. Lee SY, Lee JK. Horizontal component of partial-thickness tears of rotator cuff: imaging characteristics and comparison of ABER view with oblique coronal view at MR arthrography initial results. Radiology 2002;224(2):470–6.
38. Smith TO, Back T, Toms AP, et al. Diagnostic accuracy of ultrasound for rotator cuff tears in adults: a systematic review and meta-analysis. Clin Radiol 2011; 66(11):1036–48.
39. Wiener SN, Seitz WH Jr. Sonography of the shoulder in patient with tears of the rotator cuff: accuracy and value for selecting surgical options. AJR Am J Roentgenol 1993;160:103–7.
40. Rudzki JR, Shaffer B. New approaches to diagnosis and arthroscopic management of partial-thickness cuff tears. Clin Sports Med 2008;27:691–717.
41. Burkart SS, Diaz Pagan JL, Wirth MA, et al. Cyclic loading of anchor-based rotator cuff repairs: confirmation of the tension overload phenomenon and comparison of suture anchor fixation with transosseous fixation. Arthroscopy 1997;13:720–4.
42. Park MC, ElAttrache NS. Treating full-thickness cuff tears in the athlete: advances in arthroscopic techniques. Clin Sports Med 2008;27:719–29.
43. Curtis AS, Burbank KM, Tierney JJ, et al. The insertional footprint of the rotator cuff: an anatomic study. Arthroscopy 2006;22:603–9.
44. Minagawa H, Itoi E, Konno N, et al. Humeral attachment of the supraspinatus and infraspinatus tendons: an anatomic study. Arthroscopy 1998;14:302–6.
45. Lo KY, Burkhart SS. Transtendon arthroscopic repair of partial-thickness, articular surface tears f the rotator cuff. Arthroscopy 2004;20(2):214–20.
46. Brockmeier SF, Dodson CC, Gamradt SC, et al. Arthroscopic intratendinous repair of the delaminated partial-thickness rotator cuff tear in overhead athletes. Arthroscopy 2008;24(8):961–5.
47. Conway JE. Arthroscopic repair of partial-thickness rotator cuff tears and SLAP lesions in professional baseball players. Orthop Clin North Am 2001;32:443–56.
48. Weber SC. Arthroscopic debridement and acromioplasty versus mini-open repair in the treatment of significant partial-thickness rotator cuff tears. Arthroscopy 1999;15:126–31.
49. Budoff JE, Nirschl RP, Guidi EJ. Debridement of partial-thickness tears of the rotator cuff without acromioplasty. Long-term follow-up and review of the literature. J bone Joint Surg Am 1998;80:733–48.
50. Snyder SJ, Pachelli AF, Del Pizzo W, et al. Partial thickness rotator cuff tears: results of arthroscopic treatment. Arthroscopy 1991;7:1–7.
51. Cordasco FA, Backer M, Craig EV, et al. The partial-thickness rotator cuff tear: is acromioplasty without repair sufficient? Am J Sports Med 2002;30:257–60.
52. Payne LZ, Altchek DW, Craig EV, et al. Arthroscopic treatment of partial rotator cuff tears in young athletes. A preliminary report. Am J Sports Med 1997;25: 299–305.
53. Andrews JR, Broussard TS, Carson WG. Arthroscopy of the shoulder in the management of partial tears of the rotator cuff: a preliminary report. Arthroscopy 1985;1:117–22.
54. Reynolds SB, Dugas JR, Cain EL, et al. Debridement of small partial-thickness rotator cuff tears in elite overhead throwers. Clin Orthop Relat Res 2008;466(3): 614–21.
55. Wright SA, Cofield RH. Management of partial-thickness rotator cuff tears. J Shoulder Elbow Surg 1996;5(6):458–66.
56. Deutsch A. Arthroscopic repair of partial-thickness rotator cuff tears of the rotator cuff. J Shoulder Elbow Surg 2007;16:193–201.

57. Shin SJ. A comparison of 2 repair techniques for partial-thickness articular-sided rotator cuff tears. Arthroscopy 2012;28(1):25–33.
58. Ide J, Maeda S, Takagi K. Arthroscopic transtendon repair of partial-thickness articular-side tears of the rotator cuff: anatomical and clinical study. Am J Sports Med 2005;33:1672–9.
59. Waibl B, Buess E. Technical note: partial-thickness articular surface supraspinatus tears: a new transtendon suture technique. Arthroscopy 2005;21(3):376–81.
60. Tibone JE, Elrod B, Jobe FW, et al. Surgical treatment of tears of the rotator cuff in athletes. J Bone Joint Surg Am 1986;68:887–91.
61. Mazoue CG, Andrews JR. Repair of full-thickness rotator cuff tears in professional baseball players. Am J Sports Med 2006;34:182–9.

Failed Rotator Cuff Surgery, Evaluation and Decision Making

Scott R. Montgomery, MD, Frank A. Petrigliano, MD,
Seth C. Gamradt, MD*

KEYWORDS

- Failed rotator cuff • Rotator cuff re-tear • Revision rotator cuff repair
- Rotator cuff repair

KEY POINTS

- Recurrent or persistent tears are common after rotator cuff repair.
- The causes of failed rotator cuff surgery include biologic factors, technical errors, and traumatic failure.
- Evaluation and decision making in this difficult patient population includes a thorough history, physical examination, and appropriate imaging.
- Successful revision rotator cuff repair is most likely in younger patients with minimal muscle atrophy and tendon retraction, good preoperative forward elevation, an intact deltoid, and no evidence of cuff tear arthropathy.

INTRODUCTION

Rotator cuff repair is performed with increased frequency each year in the United States.[1,2] The purpose of rotator cuff surgery is to decrease or eliminate shoulder pain and to restore function and strength. Although subjective clinical outcomes are generally good with rotator cuff repair, a significant number of rotator cuff repairs do not demonstrate radiographic healing. In fact, persistent tears or re-tears after rotator cuff repair have been seen in up to 35% of small tears[3–7] and in as high as 94% of larger multitendon tears.[8,9] Although many patients report pain relief despite the radiographic presence of a persistent tear or re-tear, others have significant pain and disability, requiring further management. This article discusses the pathophysiology of failed rotator cuff repair and common mechanisms of failure, patient evaluation, and the treatment algorithm in the setting of failed rotator cuff surgery.

Department of Orthopaedic Surgery, David Geffen School of Medicine at UCLA, 10833 Le Conte Avenue, CHS Room 76-143, Los Angeles, CA 90095, USA
* Corresponding author.
E-mail address: sgamradt@mednet.ucla.edu

Clin Sports Med 31 (2012) 693–712
http://dx.doi.org/10.1016/j.csm.2012.07.006
0278-5919/12/$ – see front matter © 2012 Elsevier Inc. All rights reserved.

PATHOPHYSIOLOGY

A significant arm of orthopedic research has been focused on understanding the biology of the rotator cuff. Both a weakened postrepair insertion site and diminished blood flow to the rotator cuff tendon may contribute to failure. Animal studies have demonstrated that the normal rotator cuff insertion is composed of 4 distinct zones: tendon, unmineralized fibrocartilage, mineralized fibrocartilage, and bone.[10] After repair, fibrovascular scar tissue is formed between tendon and bone, resulting in a biomechanically inferior construct compared with the native enthesis.[11] Most research on this topic has been performed in animal models and few studies exist evaluating the biology of the rotator cuff in humans in vivo. Contrast-enhanced ultrasound has suggested that blood supply to the rotator cuff may affect healing. First, in the intact rotator cuff, the blood supply to the rotator cuff decreases with age, especially in those patients older than 40 years (the patient population most often undergoing repair).[12] In a second contrast-enhanced ultrasound study, Gamradt and colleagues[13] found that at 3 months after arthroscopic repair, the healing tendon is relatively avascular, whereas a significant portion of the blood supply to the healing rotator cuff originates from bone.

Although the application of growth factors, platelet-rich plasma, and synthetic grafts have been tested in animal models and in some human clinical trials, modification of surgical technique has been the primary means investigated to overcome the weakened enthesis observed after rotator cuff repair. For example, there has been a recent trend toward double row repairs and "trans-osseous equivalent" repairs, which have been found to be superior to single-row repairs in cadaveric time-zero biomechanical studies.[14] Improved radiographic tendon healing has also been observed clinically in double-row repairs.[15–17] Similarly, attempts to improve single-row repair have been made by increasing the number of fixation points with triple-loaded anchors and modifying stitch configuration to reduce cutout.[18] Disadvantages to double row repairs have also been documented, including failure at the musculotendinous junction and medial to the repair,[19] as well as theoretical restriction of blood supply to an already tenuous vascular supply to the tendon.[20] To date, clinical outcomes in randomized trials comparing double-row versus single-row rotator cuff repairs have been equivalent.[15,17] However, the vast majority of these studies have been underpowered or consist of a variety of double-row techniques that may not restore the footprint via a suture-linking construct.

MECHANISM OF FAILURE OF ROTATOR CUFF REPAIR

Determining the reason for failure of initial rotator cuff repair is an important step in deciding the most appropriate management. Rotator cuff repair failure is often multifactorial, but 3 broad mechanisms of failure exist: biologic factors, technical errors, and traumatic failure. The causes of failed rotator cuff tear are summarized in **Box 1**.

Biologic Factors

Unique biologic factors related to the patient and the anatomy of the initial tear likely contribute most to rotator cuff failure. Patient age, medical comorbidities (eg, diabetes), and tobacco use have all been implicated in failure of rotator cuff repair. Increased patient age has been shown by several authors to decrease healing rates after rotator cuff repair,[3,4,21–25] which is likely in part related to the decreased microcirculation of the tendon observed in older patients. Factors related to the tear itself have also been indicated in failure, including the initial tear size,[3,4,6,23–29] the number of tendons torn,[3] and the quality of the tendon. Nho and colleagues[24] found that the risk of a persistent tear after repair is twofold for each centimeter increase in tear size.

Box 1
Causes of failure of rotator cuff repair

1. Biologic
   a. Patient age
   b. Size of tear
   c. Fatty infiltration/Muscle atrophy
   d. Diabetes
   e. Nicotine
   f. Stiffness
2. Technical
   a. Inadequate fixation
   b. Inadequate visualization
   c. Inadequate mobilization of tear
   d. Failure of deltoid repair
   e. Improper or aggressive rehabilitation
3. Traumatic
   a. Early: Before complete cuff healing
   b. Late: Failure of a previously well-functioning repair

Fatty infiltration of the rotator cuff and the presence of muscle atrophy have received significant attention as poor prognostic factors in rotator cuff surgery. The amount of fatty infiltration present on preoperative imaging studies is often described by using the Goutallier classification,[30] which describes 5 grades: grade 0, no fatty deposit; grade 1, some fatty streaks; grade 2, more muscle than fat; grade 3, muscle equals fat; and grade 4, less muscle than fat. These changes make initial rotator cuff repair difficult and may be irreversible, even after successful rotator cuff repair; however, atrophy and fatty infiltration as assessed by magnetic resonance imaging (MRI) progress significantly more postoperatively in patients with a persistent tear compared with those with a healed repair.[31–33] Fatty infiltration of the rotator cuff also increases with the chronicity of the tear. It has been shown that moderate supraspinatus fatty infiltration appears an average of 3 years after onset of symptoms whereas severe fatty infiltration is seen roughly 5 years after the onset of shoulder symptoms.[34]

In addition to affecting the quality of repairable tissue, the fatty infiltration and muscle atrophy affects the compliance of the musculotendinous unit and thus increases tension on the repair site. This has been confirmed clinically[35] and in animal models.[36,37] In a sheep model of infraspinatus tear, earlier repair of the tendon resulted in a more rapid recovery of both muscle function and tendon elasticity, suggesting that delayed repairs may not reach the postoperative muscle function that earlier repairs can achieve.[38] In fact, clinical studies have found that earlier repair after acute rotator cuff injury results in improved clinical results when compared with a delayed repair.[39] Last, medical comorbidities, such as diabetes,[40–42] and use of tobacco inhibit healing of the rotator cuff.[43,44]

Technical Considerations

Although many factors contribute to persistent tears or re-tear after repair, there are important technical considerations that can contribute to the success or failure of initial rotator cuff repair. Surgeon volume has been found to be an independent risk factor for reoperation after rotator cuff repair.[42] Specific technical considerations that require significant attention include visualization of the entire rotator cuff, mobilization of the torn tendons, and addressing additional pathology that may affect the repaired cuff or contribute to postoperative pain.

Open, mini-open, or arthroscopic approaches have all been described for initial repair. Regardless of approach, adequate visualization of the tear is critical. Advantages of arthroscopic repair include excellent visualization of all areas of the cuff using posterior, lateral, and anterior portals, while preserving the deltoid insertion. Open repair also provides excellent visualization, but care must be taken to securely repair the deltoid. Common errors related to poor visualization include using a "mini-open" deltoid splitting approach to repair large or massive tears. The small deltoid window does not typically provide sufficient visualization of these larger tears when compared with open or arthroscopic approaches. Also, failure to expose and visualize the posterior extent of a tear can compromise arthroscopic repair of large tears. This can be seen on postoperative imaging in which fixation devices are present only in the anterior greater tuberosity in a shoulder that clearly had a large to massive tear preoperatively.

The torn rotator cuff tendon is often retracted and may have significant adhesions. The tendon must be adequately mobilized to ensure a tension-free repair. Adhesions may be present on both the bursal and articular sides of the cuff in chronic tears. Even if there is sufficient visualization and mobilization of the tendon being repaired, adequate fixation is required to avoid failure. Knot security, knotless anchor security, suture type, suture configuration, and anchor fixation in bone are all potential areas for technical failure. Cummins and Murrell[45] demonstrated that the predominant mode of failure of rotator cuff repair performed with suture anchors is sutures pulling through tendon. To prevent failure at the tendon-suture interface, the use of mattress sutures with linkage between medial and lateral rows can be used if tear configuration and tissue mobility permit.[16]

Rotator cuff tears result from a combination of intrinsic degeneration of the tendon and from extrinsic mechanical wear secondary to acromial spurs. Inadequate acromioplasty can contribute to failure of rotator cuff surgery, particularly in those patients with abnormal acromial morphology or calcification of the coracoacromial ligament. Although randomized studies have not shown a consistent clinical benefit from acromioplasty in conjunction with rotator cuff repair, untouched acromial spurs, partially resected acromial spurs, and fraying of the coracoacromial ligament indicative of impingement are common findings at the time of revision rotator cuff repair.[46,47] Djurasovic and colleagues[48] found evidence of inadequate acromioplasty at the time of revision surgery in two-thirds of their series of 80 revision rotator cuff repairs.

Traumatic Failure

Trauma can contribute to failure of rotator cuff repair. Traumatic failure can occur before complete healing of the repair, or at a later time point after the initial repair has healed and a return to function and strength has been observed. In early failures, the patient will typically report initially doing well before an event or setback, such as a fall on the arm or aggressive physical therapy. Early, aggressive postoperative rehabilitation is discouraged and may result in structural failure of the repair.[49] Surgeons, patients, and physical therapists must keep in mind that maturation of the repaired rotator cuff takes roughly 3 to 4 months[50] and thus adherence to a conservative rehabilitation protocol is important to avoid failure of the repair. In the case of a late traumatic rupture, the patient has had a previously well-functioning cuff repair with documented return of strength and range of motion and then sustains a new re-injury. A thorough workup, including history, physical examination, and imaging, is required to determine which of the aforementioned factors contributed to the failure of the rotator cuff repair and if the patient with failed cuff surgery would benefit from another operation.

EVALUATION OF THE PATIENT WITH A FAILED ROTATOR CUFF REPAIR

Despite a propensity for clinical success in rotator cuff repair, the high rate of persistent and recurrent rotator cuff tears and compromised biology of rotator cuff healing will render a certain subset of patients with persistent symptoms of weakness and pain. A careful history, physical examination, and appropriate imaging will help identify which of these patients will benefit from further surgery and which patients should be managed nonoperatively.

History and Physical Examination

A careful history is paramount to understanding the potential causes of rotator cuff repair failure, to determine the appropriate treatment, and to define patient expectations. Important components of the history include duration of pain and date of initial injury, mechanism of injury, sports participation and occupation, complete medical history (systemic disease, diabetes, tobacco use), location and character of pain, aggravating or relieving factors, and presence of neurologic symptoms or neck pain. The patient should be asked if any improvement in symptoms was noted after the initial repair. All previous surgeries should be documented, and if a previous surgery was performed at an outside institution, the patient's medical records, including operative reports, preoperative imaging, and arthroscopic photos, should be acquired and reviewed. The postoperative rehabilitation protocol and duration of immobilization should also be noted.

Physical examination begins with careful inspection of the shoulder with comparison to the contralateral side. Location and healing of portals or incisions from prior surgeries should be examined for healing, contracture, inflammation, erythema, or tenderness. Infection is relatively rare after rotator cuff repair, but must be ruled in the evaluation of failed repair. Patients with infection often complain of constant pain as opposed to intermittent, activity-related pain associated with rotator cuff dysfunction. Propionobacterium acnes has been the most commonly identified bacteria after rotator cuff repair, present in 50% to 86% of postoperative infections.[51,52] Diagnosis is critical, as treatment requires surgical irrigation and debridement and intravenous antibiotics.

Deformity or atrophy of the deltoid or rotator cuff should be documented. Poor preoperative deltoid function is a poor prognostic sign for revision rotator cuff repair.[48] The status of the subscapularis tendon, acromioclavicular joint, and long head of the biceps tendon (popeye sign or tenderness to palpation) must be examined to identify other pain generators and concomitant pathology to be addressed at the time of revision surgery. Range-of-motion testing is performed, including active and passive forward elevation, external rotation, and internal rotation. Range of motion is frequently preserved in patients with smaller tears and pain may be elicited only at extreme flexion or rotation. Patients with large and massive tears are most likely to lose active range of motion. Passive range of motion is assessed to rule out postoperative adhesive capsulitis or progression to arthritis.

Muscle strength testing of the deltoid, supraspinatus, subscapularis, and external rotation is performed and compared with the contralateral side. Muscle strength testing has increased importance in the revision setting, as less accurate information is obtained with MRI. This is particularly true for the subscapularis; bear-hug, belly-press, and lift-off tests are all performed. There is also evidence that physical examination maneuvers can provide information about tear size[53] and fatty infiltration.[54] A positive external rotation lag sign, in which external rotation cannot be maintained in 20° of abduction and maximum external rotation, yields a 65% sensitivity for detecting tears extending into the infraspinatus tendon. Muscle testing is followed by Neer and Hawkins impingement signs. Importantly, the Spurling test is performed to rule out cervical radiculopathy masquerading as shoulder pain.

Imaging

Plain radiographs are the initial imaging modality used in revision rotator cuff surgery. Anteroposterior, Grashey, axillary, and Y views of the affected shoulder are performed and assessed for the following factors: status of the acromioclavicular (AC) joint (normal, osteoarthritis [OA], resected), presence of acromial spur, presence of inferior AC osteophytes, status of greater tuberosity (previous trough, anchor placement), presence of joint space narrowing or osteophytes indicative of OA, assessment of acromio-humeral interval, and presence of a high-riding humeral head. It is important to look for evidence of rotator cuff arthropathy (fixed high-riding humeral head and arthritis), which are contraindications to revision rotator cuff repair. However, isolated proximal migration of the humeral head is not necessarily a contraindication to revision repair and can improve following repair.[55]

Although MRI is now the gold standard for imaging the rotator cuff, its accuracy is diminished in the postoperative setting. The sensitivity appears to remain high (91%) in the diagnosis of persistent tears, but the specificity of MRI in this setting has been reported to be 25%, which can result in the overdiagnosis of re-tears.[56] Surgical implants, such as suture anchors, can also result in the generation of artifact, although identifying the number and location of suture anchors, as well as the adjacent bone quality in the greater tuberosity is valuable for operative planning. Despite these limitations, valuable information regarding the state of the rotator cuff can be obtained with MRI, and a recent noncontrast MRI is preferred to evaluate a patient's shoulder after rotator cuff repair. If possible, the patient's MRI from before the first surgery should be reviewed for comparison to help determine the mechanism of surgical failure. Gadolinium-enhanced MRI can certainly be used, but it is not routinely necessary.

MRI is currently the primary means to assess reparability of the rotator cuff after failed repair. Davidson and Burkhart[26] have recently published a classification system to correlate rotator cuff tear pattern with prognosis after repair. Two factors help determine the reparability of the tear: the degree of muscle atrophy on sagittal views through the rotator cuff muscle bellies at the level of the scapula, and the amount of retraction on coronal views, which can be measured in relation to its proximity to the previous trough or anchor sites in the greater tuberosity. It is reasonable to attempt revision rotator cuff repair if the apex of the tendon is lateral to the glenohumeral joint on the coronal plain and if the Goutallier classifaction is stage 3 or better (muscle equals fat). However, fatty infiltration of the cuff is not an absolute contraindication to revision cuff surgery.[57]

Ultrasound can also be an effective adjunct in evaluating the integrity of the rotator cuff postoperatively. When compared with revision arthroscopic surgical findings, ultrasound demonstrated a sensitivity of 91%, specificity of 86%, and accuracy of 89% for detection of postoperative cuff integrity.[58] Computed tomography arthrography is also useful for evaluating the rotator cuff, but because of high radiation exposure from this procedure, it has largely been replaced by MRI and is primarily reserved for patients with a contraindication to MRI, such as a pacemaker.

RESULTS OF REVISION ROTATOR CUFF REPAIR

Several case series have reported outcomes after open and arthroscopic revision rotator cuff repair (**Table 1**). Success has been achieved with both open and arthroscopic techniques; however, it is clear from reviewing these studies that patient selection is critical in predicting success of repair. The largest published series of open revision cuff repairs was performed by Djurasovic and colleagues[48] and the Shoulder Service at Columbia University. In 80 patients undergoing revision rotator cuff repair, these investigators found the following factors most important in obtaining successful outcomes: (1) intact deltoid, (2) good rotator cuff tissue, (3) preoperative active elevation past 90°, (4) only one previous surgery.

Arthroscopic revision rotator cuff repair has also been proven to be effective in the treatment of failed rotator cuff repair. Keener and colleagues,[25] Lo and Burkhart,[47] Piasecki and colleagues,[46] and Ladermann and colleagues have all documented in retrospective case series that arthroscopic revision rotator cuff repair is clinically effective in most cases in improving pain and function. Most recently, Ladermann and colleagues[61] published a series of 74 arthroscopic revision rotator cuff repairs, in which 21 were nonmassive, defined as tears measuring less than 5 cm in the anterior-to-posterior dimension, and 53 were massive tears (greater than 5 cm). No significant difference in patients with nonmassive compared with massive tears was observed in postoperative forward elevation, pain, or functional outcome. Poor functional outcomes were associated with female gender, preoperative active forward flexion less than 136°, and increased preoperative pain score.

INDICATIONS FOR REVISION REPAIR

Several factors are considered to determine if a patient with a failed rotator cuff repair would benefit from further surgery (**Box 2**). The most favorable candidate for revision rotator cuff repair would be a relatively young patient with high functional demand, a reparable tear without atrophy (**Fig. 1**), good preoperative range of motion, an intact deltoid, and only one prior surgery. Unfortunately, these candidates are in the minority. As a result, nonoperative treatment is typically the most appropriate management of patients with a failed rotator cuff repair. It is important to have a frank discussion with patients who are not good revision candidates. The indications for debridement, latissimus transfer, allograft augmentation, and reverse arthroplasty are beyond the scope of this review but have been comprehensively reviewed previously.[40] If a patient is not a good revision candidate, continued rehabilitation is prescribed, with a focus on Levy anterior deltoid strengthening exercises.[62]

Using the criteria in **Box 2**, if a dedicated course of physical therapy fails, we offer revision rotator cuff repair to those patients with painful, full-thickness tears that appear reparable on MRI. Often, the most satisfying revisions are those cases in which technical error or trauma has caused failure of cuff surgery in a patient with good-quality rotator cuff tissue. Reattempting repair on a tear that was borderline reparable at the index surgery because of muscle atrophy is typically unsatisfying.

SURGICAL TECHNIQUE

The preoperative discussion with the patient is critical to the success of a revision rotator cuff repair. The surgeon needs to formally educate the patient about his or

Table 1
Outcomes following open and arthroscopic revision rotator cuff repair

Author	No. of Shoulders	Mean Age, y	Mean Follow-Up, mo	Mean Time to Revision, mo	Outcome Measures	Results	Factors Associated with Improved Outcomes
Open Revision Rotator Cuff Repair							
Bigliani et al,[59] 1992	31	57	75	13	Rated as excellent, good, fair, or poor based on pain, ROM, and function	Excellent 19%, Good 32%, Fair 23%, Poor 26%	1. Intact acromion 2. Intact deltoid origin 3. Tissue quality at time of revision
DeOrio et al,[60] 1984	27	52	64	46	Rated as good, fair, or poor based on pain, motion, strength, patient's response, and need for additional surgery	Good 17%, Fair 25%, Poor 58%	1. Functioning deltoid 2. Smaller cuff tear found at revision 3. Less tissue needed to close tendon defect
Djurasovic et al,[48] 2001	80	59	49	6.5	Rated as excellent, good, fair, or poor based on pain, ROM, and function	Excellent 33%, Good 25%, Fair 11%, Poor 31%	1. Intact deltoid origin 2. Tissue quality at time of revision 3. Preoperative active elevation of >90° 4. Only one prior procedure
Neviaser,[49] 1997	50	54.5	30	16.9	Pain, active elevation, patient satisfaction	92% improvement in pain, 8% pain unchanged; 26 patients improved average of 50°, 22 remained unchanged, 2 lost motion; 90% satisfaction rate	1. Intact deltoid 2. Adequate decompression 3. Closure of all defects with tendon-to-bone junctures 4. No weights or resistive exercises during the first 3 mo postoperatively

Arthroscopic Revision Rotator Cuff Repair

Study	N	Mean age	Follow-up	Outcome measures	Results	Prognostic factors
Keener et al,[25] 2010	21	55.6	33	Visual Analog Pain Scale, SST, ASES score	VAS improved from 6.1 to 2.8; SST improved from 5.3 to 8.8; ASES improved from 40.1 to 73.0	1. Younger age 2. Fewer tendons involved 3. Intact repair at time of revision
Ladermann et al,[61] 2011	74	59.2 nonmassive, 61.5 massive	44.3 nonmassive, 48.0 massive	UCLA score, ASES Score, VAS pain score, Single Assessment Numeric Evaluation	Active forward flexion improved 135.6°–152.1°, pain score improved from 4.9 to 1.9, UCLA score increased from 17.1 to 15.9, ASES increased from 47.1 to 75.4	1. Male gender 2. Preoperative forward flexion greater than 136° 3. Preoperative pain score below 5 points
Lo and Burkhart,[47] 2004	14	57.9	23.4	UCLA score	Mean 13.1 preoperatively to mean 28.6 postoperatively	1. Intact deltoid 2. Visualization and classification of all tears (improved with arthroscopy)
Piasecki et al,[46] 2010	54	54.9	31.1	Visual Analog Pain Scale, SST, ASES score	VAS improved from 5.17 to 2.75; SST improved from 3.6 to 7.5; ASES improved from 43.8 to 68.1	1. Male gender 2. Only one prior procedure

Abbreviations: ASES, American Shoulder and Elbow Score; ROM, range of motion; SST, Simple Shoulder Test; UCLA, University of California Los Angeles; VAS, Visual Analog Scale.

> **Box 2**
> **Factors influencing the decision to revise a failed rotator cuff repair**
>
> - Reparability of tear (based on recent MRI showing level of muscle atrophy and retraction of tendon)
> - Active range of motion (preoperative forward elevation of less than 90° is a poor prognostic sign)
> - Status of deltoid muscle (a poor deltoid predicts poor results)
> - Number of surgeries (more than one surgery is a poor prognostic sign)
> - Confirmed attempt at a strict rehabilitation protocol
> - Functional demands
> - Pain level

her condition and set the patient's expectations at an appropriate level. Inflated patient expectations will compromise the outcome of the surgery. For example, a patient with a massive retracted recurrent rotator cuff tear that is expecting full, unrestricted return to activity does not have an understanding of the severity of the condition being treated. A patient must demonstrate an understanding of the severity of the condition, the goals of the revision surgery, and the possible complications that can occur with revision repair.

Dr Edward Craig and Dr Robert Bell have both published the content of their preoperative discussion for rotator cuff repair and these discussions are relevant in the revision setting.[63,64] For revision repair, the following points are emphasized: the primary reason to have rotator cuff surgery is to decrease pain, whereas added function is an additional benefit and the shoulder will not likely return to "normal." Additionally, revision repairs have a high likelihood of re-tearing again and some patients with large tears will develop arthritis (rotator cuff tear arthropathy) in the future. Although there is a possibility that a second attempt at repair may not improve pain or function, because the repair is being performed arthroscopically, there is only a small chance of being made worse. The rehabilitation will consist of at least 4 to 6 weeks of healing in a sling, 6 weeks passive range of motion, 6 weeks active range of motion, and

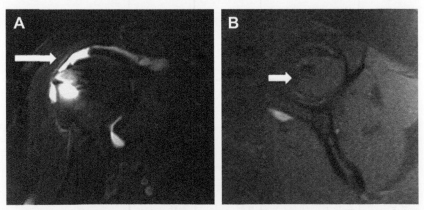

Fig. 1. (A) A 50-year-old woman status post 1-anchor rotator cuff repair 4 years prior with MRI evidence of re-tear (*arrow*) on coronal MRI and (B) minimal fatty infiltration on sagittal MRI.

6 weeks of strengthening. Pain and stiffness can persist for as long as 6 months and continued improvement can be seen in shoulders until 1 year.

Last, in the preoperative workup we are certain to evaluate both the AC joint and biceps tendon to determine their contribution to the patient's symptoms. Concomitant biceps tendonitis or AC joint arthrosis are subsequently addressed at the time of revision rotator cuff repair.

Operating Room Setup

We prefer the beach chair position for rotator cuff surgery. Advantages of this position include the effect of gravity opening the subacromial space, effective and simple internal and external rotation of the arm to view posterior and anterior aspects of the tear, respectively, and straightforward conversion to open surgery if necessary. Lateral decubitus is also a reasonable position for rotator cuff surgery. Surgeon preference and familiarity are most important when selecting surgical position. We also perform the vast majority of revision repairs arthroscopically. We favor double row repairs with suture anchors, knot tying, and linkage between medial and lateral row, if possible. However, a single-row repair to the medial aspect of the footprint is performed if a double-row repair results in excessive tension on the tendon. Although newer knotless designs provide excellent and secure repairs in mobile, crescent-shaped tears, we do not believe that they are versatile enough to be used effectively in every revision case.

As outlined in **Table 1**, direct comparison of arthroscopic versus open revision repairs in the literature is impossible owing to difference of techniques, disparity of patient populations, and inconsistency of tear size. Surgeon preference and familiarity remains the most important consideration in choosing between the two. Early morbidity secondary to the incision will be experienced after an open revision cuff repair, but functional outcomes are likely to be similar if the deltoid is sufficiently repaired. If a patient has a large, retracted tear, it is possible that the cuff will not be adequately mobilized arthroscopically and the patient should be informed of the possibility of converting to an open procedure. We feel that the arthroscopic approach is slightly safer than an open approach because it carries minimal risk of compromising a functioning deltoid. We do not recommend treating massive tears via a "mini-open" approach because of the limited visualization through the deltoid split.

At our institution, an ultrasound-guided interscalene block is performed by a regional anesthesiologist followed by general anesthesia or sedation. The patient is placed in the beach chair postion at 60 to 70° using an operating table with a beach chair head positioner. Ideally, the systolic blood pressure is maintained between 95 and 110 mm Hg to ensure cerebral perfusion while limiting subacromial bleeding. Adding of 1 mL of 1:1000 epinephrine per 3000 mL of arthroscopy fluid may also improve hemostasis. An arthroscopic pump, set initially at 35 mm Hg, is typically used to improve visualization. The entire arm is then prepped and placed in a Spider arm positioner (Tenet Medical, Calgary, Alberta, Canada) after easy access to the posterior and anterior shoulder is confirmed. Distraction of the subacromial space and flexible adjustment of internal and external rotation are allowed with a Spider arm. The arm is not abducted for the repair so that tension on the repair can be truly assessed. The following instrumentation is required: 5 mm cannula, 8.25 mm cannula, suture retriever, arthroscopic grasper, knot pusher, devices for antegrade and retrograde suture passage, and suture anchors of choice for medial and lateral double row repair. For antegrade suture passage, we prefer the Expressew suture passer (Depuy-Mitek, Raynham, MA) or an equivalent device.

Portals

Portal placement is critical for efficient and successful revision rotator cuff repair. Placement should not be influenced by portals created during prior surgery. The posterior viewing portal is more superior and more lateral than for cases that are predominately glenohumeral. Preferably, this portal is placed 1 cm inferior and 1 cm medial to the posterolateral acromion. This is a suboptimal portal for extensive glenohumeral work, but it then allows for improved visualization of the tear in the subacromial space. Spinal needle localization is used for remaining portals, which include the anterior portal (localized mid acromion anteriorly) and the lateral portal (localized in the center of the tear laterally). After insertion of the arthroscope, we place a rotator interval portal anteriorly. Attention is paid to staying lateral on the skin so the portal functions well for subsequent subacromial arthroscopy.

Diagnostic Arthroscopy, Rotator Cuff Repair, and Associated Procedures

A standard diagnostic arthroscopy is performed, with a focus on assessing the biceps tendon, subscapularis, and evaluating the size of the supraspinatus/infraspinatus tear. An efficient but thorough analysis of the glenohumeral portion is needed before advancing to the subacromial space. If indicated, a biceps tenotomy or biceps tenodesis is performed. The long head of the biceps must be discussed preoperatively with each patient to determine the patient's preference. To include the gamut of pathology that can be encountered during revision repair, the description that follows describes a repair of a massive tear with involvement of subscapularis, supraspinatus, and part of the infraspinatus.

Most commonly, subscapularis tears in this setting involve only the upper half of the tendon and can be repaired with the arthroscope in the glenohumeral joint. Second portal placement through a torn supraspinatus tear aids subscapularis repair. The medial sling of the biceps (referred to as the "comma" tissue by Burkhart and Tehrany[55]) is used to identify the superolateral boarder of the subscapularis. The lateral portal is placed through the supraspinatus tear and the anterior portal is placed just above the subscapularis and medial to the comma tissue. A traction stitch is placed in the tendon using the Expressew and placed outside the cannula through the lateral portal. Adhesions are cleared using radiofrequency using traction on the tendon via the lateral portal. This is complete when the tendon can easily be reduced to the lesser tuberosity. It is critical to remove soft tissue anterior to the tendon so that sutures can be passed low and medial in the tendon under direct vision. The arthroscope is then driven over the top of the humeral head and the camera is pointed directly inferiorly to visualize the lesser tuberosity. A 70° arthroscope can be used to improve visualization of the lesser tuberosity, but is not typically necessary. The lesser tuberosity is then gently decorticated and a double-loaded suture anchor is placed through the anterior portal. Directing the surgeon's hand toward the patient's face facilitates the appropriate angle of anchor placement. Flexing and slightly externally rotating the shoulder also assists proper anchor placement. The Expressew is then used to place a low mattress stitch and a high simple stitch in the subscapularis tendon. Suture passage is accomplished from the lateral portal, passing the limb of suture from posterior to anterior through the tendon and retrieving each limb through the anterior portal. The arm is then internally rotated slightly to decrease tension and the knots are tied arthroscopically. We prefer to tie arthroscopic knots with half hitches as we use mostly mattress sutures and therefore rarely use sliding knots.

Following subscapularis repair, we prefer to mobilize the articular side of the supraspinatus/infraspinatus tear while in the glenohumeral joint, which is technically easier compared with having the arthroscope in the subacromial space. Starting anteriorly, we release just above the glenoid in the plane between labrum and rotator cuff using radiofrequency. The coracoid process is the anterior limit of the release. Additionally, care should be taken to avoid releasing beyond 2 cm medial to the glenoid to avoid injury to the suprascapular nerve. The release is carried as far posteriorly as necessary.

After the articular-sided cuff release, the arthroscope is removed and carefully reintroduced into the subacromial space with attention to staying in the plane above bursa. A complete subacromial bursectomy is then performed. In the revision setting, previous surgical scarring will be present, making it difficult to distinguish rotator cuff and bursal tissue. The rotator cuff should be identified anteriorly first and then the bursectomy directed posteriorly with the shaver facing away from rotator cuff. Goals of bursectomy are twofold. First, the entirety of the rotator cuff tear must be visualized, which requires identifying the extent of the tear anteriorly and where the cuff inserts posteriorly on the humeral head. Second, the bursectomy is critical to visualizing stitches that are to be placed in the posterior cuff. After completing the bursectomy and establishing the tear pattern, we develop a plan for fixing the tear arthroscopically. It is helpful to view the tear from at least 2 orthogonal portals to plan the repair. We prefer to place the camera in the lateral portal intermittently to garner a "50-yard-line" view of the tear.

The mobility of the tear is assessed by grasping the rotator cuff from both laterally and anteriorly to test its excursion and the ability to reduce it to the greater tuberosity. In large tears, the tissue is typically more mobile from posterior to anterior than it is from medial to lateral. A bursal-sided release using radiofrequency is then performed first without traction on the rotator cuff and then a second time with 2 traction stitches pulling the tendon from medial to lateral. In large tears, an anterior interval slide can be performed. We commonly release back to the scapular spine. During the release, bleeding is often incited, particularly posterior and medially. If a large bleeder is encountered it is best to keep the arthroscope directly at the site of bleeding and then bring the cautery device to the scope to avoid high pump pressures and "red-out" situations. Once maximum excursion of the rotator cuff is obtained, we have an assistant hold gentle traction on the rotator cuff during the acromioplasty to perhaps gain some extra excursion of the tendon.

After the rotator cuff has been adequately mobilized, attention is turned to the acromion. The anterolateral aspect of the acromion is identified. Using radiofrequency, soft tissue is stripped off the undersurface of the acromion moving medially and posteriorly. The entire anterior acromion and AC joint are exposed. The acromioplasty is performed using an oval burr such that the anterior acromion is flush with the posterior acromion. Avoiding the deltoid fascia and fluid extravasation is critical in this portion of the procedure. The distal clavicle is then resected in standard fashion if necessary based on history, physical examination, and preoperative radiographs.

The anterior (5.0 mm) and lateral (8.25 mm) cannulas are reestablished after the revision acromioplasty is finished. The greater tuberosity is cleared of soft tissue and then lightly decorticated using a burr. Before anchor placement, U-shaped tears and L-shaped tears are converted to crescent-shaped tears with margin convergence sutures. We prefer passing margin convergence sutures using 2 individual bites from the Expressew device. The posterior limb of suture is passed through the anterior cannula and the anterior limb of suture through the lateral cannula. These knots are tied down immediately and the tear is reassessed to determine if more margin convergence is needed.

Once the tear has been converted to a crescent-shaped pattern, we begin anchor placement with separate 5-mm stab incisions for each anchor starting posteriorly and working anteriorly. The first anchor is placed through a separate stab incision just off the lateral edge of the acromion. A blunt trocar opens the deltoid slightly and the anchor is inserted in the posterior aspect of the tear in the medial footprint of the rotator cuff. We almost always use medial footprint anchors. In shoulders with immobile tissue, single-row repairs to the medial footprint are performed, whereas double-row repairs are performed in shoulders with adequate and reducible cuff tissue. The first 1 or 2 antegrade suture passings are usually performed from the anterior cannula to reach the posterior cuff to attain the posterior to anterior mobility that is common in large tears. Typically, horizontal mattress sutures are used, spaced 5 to 7 mm apart, taking 15-mm to 18-mm bites of tissue. Once all limbs of suture are passed satisfactorily, the sutures are retrieved out the separate anchor stab, docking them without confusion until tying. In general, we use one medial row anchor for every 1.0 to 1.5 cm of tear width. Each successive anchor is placed through a separate stab incision avoiding suture confusion. Once all medial row sutures have been passed, the medial row is tied arthroscopically from posterior-to-anterior and the sutures are not cut. It is critical for the knot pusher to recreate the angle of anchor insertion during knot tying to enable close coaptation of tendon to bone. Once all knots have been tied, the sutures are all retrieved out the anterior cannula. The lateral aspect of the greater tuberosity is then cleared of soft tissue to allow for visualization for placement of the lateral row suture anchors. Sutures from the medial row are draped over the cuff edge and secured on tension inside lateral row anchors inserted in standard fashion in the greater tuberosity. Choice of implants is probably not critical. If the repair fails, it is highly unlikely that it will fail because of the strength of suture or fixation devices; it will fail because of suture cutout of poor-quality tissue. We will occasionally augment our repair with platelet-rich plasma (PRP), as per Gamradt and colleagues[65] in cases of diabetes or smoking, although there is no current level 1 evidence to support this use at this time. In addition, the indications for suprascapular nerve decompression deserve further study in this population.[66]

We prefer to close each portal with buried 4-0 monocryl stitches, mastisol, and steri-strips. This is a very cosmetic closure and saves time in the office avoiding suture removal. An abduction pillow sling and cold therapy device is placed in the operating room. In most cases, we allow immediate shoulder shrugs, distal range of motion, passive forward elevation to 90°, and passive external rotation to neutral. If a tear is particularly large or tissue quality is poor, we will completely immobilize the shoulder

---

Box 3
Summary of important consideration in surgical technique

- Use strict criteria when deciding to revise a rotator cuff surgery; most failed cuff repairs should be treated nonoperatively.

- Discuss realistic goals for surgery with patients, explain the natural history of rotator cuff disease, and inform them of the risk that their repair could fail again.

- Use a high lateral posterior portal for optimal visualization.

- Mobilize the articular side of the rotator cuff while still in the glenohumeral joint.

- Mobilize extensively on the bursal side of the tear using traction stitches to facilitate a tension-free repair.

- Assess mobility and tissue quality of each tear and individualize repair construct for each tear.

- Convert complex tears to simple ones using margin convergence sutures.

- Resist the temptation to do too much; many tears are not completely reparable.

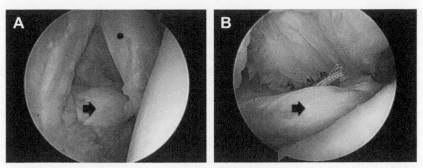

Fig. 2. (*A*) Vertical biceps (*circle*) and torn subscapularis (*arrow*) viewed from a posterior portal. (*B*) Arthroscopic view of a biceps tenotomy and subscapularis tendon (*arrow*) repair.

for no longer than 4 weeks. The sling is discontinued and active range of motion is started at week 6. Very light strengthening can be started at 12 weeks. Patients are advised that pain and stiffness can persist for 6 months and that the shoulder will continue to improve for 1 year. A summary of important points regarding surgical technique is provided in **Box 3** and relevant arthroscopic images are shown in **Figs. 2** and **3**.

ROLE OF BIOLOGICS IN REVISION ROTATOR CUFF REPAIR

Several strategies are currently being investigated to augment rotator cuff repair to decrease failure rates. These strategies include allograft, extracellular matrices (ECMs), and PRP, which have been tested clinically in humans, as well as growth factors, stem cells, and gene therapy that are currently under study in animal models. To date, application of transforming growth factor-β3,[67] platelet-derived growth factor-β,[68] fibroblast growth factor-2,[69] scleraxis[70] and membrane type 1–matrix

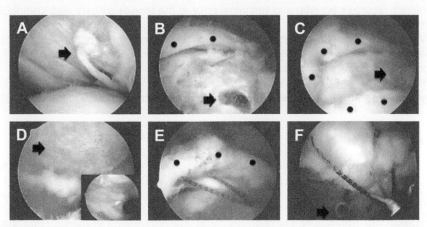

Fig. 3. (*A*) Intra-articular view of case from **Fig. 2** revealing re-tear in supraspinatus and with pull through of previous suture (*arrow*). (*B*) Subacromial view from posterior showing free cuff edge (*circles*) and previous metallic suture anchor (*arrow*). (*C*) Subacromial view after bursectomy showing U-shaped rotator cuff tear (*cuff edges marked with circles*) and greater tuberosity (*arrow*). (*D*) Residual acromial spur (*arrow*) and acromioplasty (*inset*). (*E*) After suture passage of medial row (*cuff edges marked with circles*). (*F*) Completed double-row revision rotator cuff repair after placement of lateral row suture anchors (*arrow*).

metalloproteinase[71] in animal models have improved both the histology at the rotator cuff tendon insertion site after repair and/or the biomechanical strength of the repair. Adenoviral vectors have been used to deliver some these factors via transduction of pluripotent mesenchymal stem cells. Although promising results have been seen in animal models and in vitro studies, they have not yet been tested in humans in the setting of rotator cuff repair.

Clinically available approaches include extracellular matrices, xenograft and allograft tissue, and PRP. Of these, PRP has received significant attention and is the only approach that has been evaluated in randomized prospective clinical trials. In studies performed by Randelli and colleagues,[72] Castricini and colleagues,[73] and Rodeo and colleagues,[74] no differences were found in healing rates of those rotator cuff repairs treated with PRP compared with those without PRP. Randelli and colleagues[72] found that pain level in the first month after surgery was improved in the PRP group and shoulder function and strength was improved at 3 months in the PRP group as determined by the Simple Shoulder Test, University of California Los Angeles, constant scores, and strength in external rotation. However, no difference was found at later time points, including 2-year follow-up. Although each of the strategies described herein have potential to address the biologic hurdles present in rotator cuff repair, none has yet to have a significant clinical impact.

SUMMARY

Rotator cuff repair is very likely to be clinically successful when performed well and rehabilitated properly, especially when judged with patient satisfaction outcome scores. A healed rotator cuff tendon will likely result in an improved and lasting clinical result. Recurrent tears will still be present despite optimal mobilization and fixation of the rotator cuff to bone, especially in large tears with retraction and atrophy. Failure of rotator cuff repairs is multifactorial with biologic factors, such as age, tear size, and fatty infiltration probably most critical. Other patient-related factors (ie, diabetes, smoking), recurrent trauma, and technical error at the time of surgery also contribute to rotator cuff repair failure.

When managing a patient with a symptomatic re-tear, revision rotator cuff repair can be a very successful procedure, but patient selection is critical and managing patient expectations is paramount. Ideal candidates for revision rotator cuff repair have minimal muscle atrophy, minimal tendon retracted, preoperative forward elevation of greater than 90°, a functioning deltoid, and no evidence of cuff tear arthropathy.

REFERENCES

1. Yamaguchi K. New guideline on rotator cuff problems. In: Terry Canale S, editor. AAOS Now. Rosemont (IL): American Academy of Orthopaedic Surgeons; 2011. Available at http://www.aaos.org/news/aaosnow/jan11/cover1.asp. Accessed August 20th, 2012.
2. Colvin AC, Egorova N, Harrison AK, et al. National trends in rotator cuff repair. J Bone Joint Surg Am 2012;94(3):227–33.
3. Gazielly DF, Gleyze P, Montagnon C. Functional and anatomical results after rotator cuff repair. Clin Orthop Relat Res 1994;304:43–53.
4. Harryman DT 2nd, Mack LA, Wang KY, et al. Repairs of the rotator cuff. Correlation of functional results with integrity of the cuff. J Bone Joint Surg Am 1991; 73(7):982–9.

5. Knudsen HB, Gelineck J, Sojbjerg JO, et al. Functional and magnetic resonance imaging evaluation after single-tendon rotator cuff reconstruction. J Shoulder Elbow Surg 1999;8(3):242–6.

6. Liu SH, Baker CL. Arthroscopically assisted rotator cuff repair: correlation of functional results with integrity of the cuff. Arthroscopy 1994;10(1):54–60.

7. Wulker N, Melzer C, Wirth CJ. Shoulder surgery for rotator cuff tears. Ultrasonographic 3-year follow-up of 97 cases. Acta Orthop Scand 1991;62(2):142–7.

8. Calvert PT, Packer NP, Stoker DJ, et al. Arthrography of the shoulder after operative repair of the torn rotator cuff. J Bone Joint Surg Br 1986;68(1):147–50.

9. Galatz LM, Ball CM, Teefey SA, et al. The outcome and repair integrity of completely arthroscopically repaired large and massive rotator cuff tears. J Bone Joint Surg Am 2004;86-A(2):219–24.

10. Woo SL, An KN, Arnoczky SP, et al. Anatomy, biology, and biomechanics of tendon, ligament, and meniscus. In: Sheldon RS, editor. Orthopaedic basic science. Rosemont (IL): American Academy of Orthopaedic Surgeons; 1994. p. 45–87.

11. Gulotta LV, Rodeo SA. Growth factors for rotator cuff repair. Clin Sports Med 2009; 28(1):13–23.

12. Rudzki JR, Adler RS, Warren RF, et al. Contrast-enhanced ultrasound characterization of the vascularity of the rotator cuff tendon: age- and activity-related changes in the intact asymptomatic rotator cuff. J Shoulder Elbow Surg 2008; 17(Suppl 1):96S–100S.

13. Gamradt SC, Gallo RA, Adler RS, et al. Vascularity of the supraspinatus tendon three months after repair: characterization using contrast-enhanced ultrasound. J Shoulder Elbow Surg 2010;19(1):73–80.

14. Wall LB, Keener JD, Brophy RH. Double-row vs single-row rotator cuff repair: a review of the biomechanical evidence. J Shoulder Elbow Surg 2009;18(6): 933–41.

15. Nho SJ, Slabaugh MA, Seroyer ST, et al. Does the literature support double-row suture anchor fixation for arthroscopic rotator cuff repair? A systematic review comparing double-row and single-row suture anchor configuration. Arthroscopy 2009;25(11):1319–28.

16. Burkhart SS, Cole BJ. Bridging self-reinforcing double-row rotator cuff repair: we really are doing better. Arthroscopy 2010;26(5):677–80.

17. Duquin TR, Buyea C, Bisson LJ. Which method of rotator cuff repair leads to the highest rate of structural healing? A systematic review. Am J Sports Med 2010; 38(4):835–41.

18. Castagna A, Garofalo R, Conti M, et al. Arthroscopic rotator cuff repair using a triple-loaded suture anchor and a modified Mason-Allen technique (Alex stitch). Arthroscopy 2007;23(4):440.e1–4.

19. Trantalis JN, Boorman RS, Pletsch K, et al. Medial rotator cuff failure after arthroscopic double-row rotator cuff repair. Arthroscopy 2008;24(6):727–31.

20. Accousti K, Gladstone J, Parsons B, et al. In-vivo measurement of rotator cuff perfusion using laser dopplerflowmetry. In: Programs and abstracts of the 26th Arthroscopy Association of North America Annual Meeting. San Francisco, April 26–29, 2007.

21. Boileau P, Brassart N, Watkinson DJ, et al. Arthroscopic repair of full-thickness tears of the supraspinatus: does the tendon really heal? J Bone Joint Surg Am 2005;87(6):1229–40.

22. DeFranco MJ, Bershadsky B, Ciccone J, et al. Functional outcome of arthroscopic rotator cuff repairs: a correlation of anatomic and clinical results. J Shoulder Elbow Surg 2007;16(6):759–65.

23. Cole BJ, McCarty LP 3rd, Kang RW, et al. Arthroscopic rotator cuff repair: prospective functional outcome and repair integrity at minimum 2-year follow-up. J Shoulder Elbow Surg 2007;16(5):579–85.
24. Nho SJ, Brown BS, Lyman S, et al. Prospective analysis of arthroscopic rotator cuff repair: prognostic factors affecting clinical and ultrasound outcome. J Shoulder Elbow Surg 2009;18(1):13–20.
25. Keener JD, Wei AS, Kim HM, et al. Revision arthroscopic rotator cuff repair: repair integrity and clinical outcome. J Bone Joint Surg Am 2010;92(3):590–8.
26. Davidson J, Burkhart SS. The geometric classification of rotator cuff tears: a system linking tear pattern to treatment and prognosis. Arthroscopy 2010; 26(3):417–24.
27. Bishop J, Klepps S, Lo IK, et al. Cuff integrity after arthroscopic versus open rotator cuff repair: a prospective study. J Shoulder Elbow Surg 2006;15(3):290–9.
28. Huijsmans PE, Pritchard MP, Berghs BM, et al. Arthroscopic rotator cuff repair with double-row fixation. J Bone Joint Surg Am 2007;89(6):1248–57.
29. Sugaya H, Maeda K, Matsuki K, et al. Repair integrity and functional outcome after arthroscopic double-row rotator cuff repair. A prospective outcome study. J Bone Joint Surg Am 2007;89(5):953–60.
30. Goutallier D, Postel JM, Bernageau J, et al. Fatty muscle degeneration in cuff ruptures. Pre- and postoperative evaluation by CT scan. Clin Orthop Relat Res 1994;304:78–83.
31. Gerber C, Schneeberger AG, Hoppeler H, et al. Correlation of atrophy and fatty infiltration on strength and integrity of rotator cuff repairs: a study in thirteen patients. J Shoulder Elbow Surg 2007;16(6):691–6.
32. Gladstone JN, Bishop JY, Lo IK, et al. Fatty infiltration and atrophy of the rotator cuff do not improve after rotator cuff repair and correlate with poor functional outcome. Am J Sports Med 2007;35(5):719–28.
33. Liem D, Lichtenberg S, Magosch P, et al. Magnetic resonance imaging of arthroscopic supraspinatus tendon repair. J Bone Joint Surg Am 2007;89(8):1770–6.
34. Melis B, DeFranco MJ, Chuinard C, et al. Natural history of fatty infiltration and atrophy of the supraspinatus muscle in rotator cuff tears. Clin Orthop Relat Res 2010;468(6):1498–505.
35. Hersche O, Gerber C. Passive tension in the supraspinatus musculotendinous unit after long-standing rupture of its tendon: a preliminary report. J Shoulder Elbow Surg 1998;7(4):393–6.
36. Gimbel JA, Mehta S, Van Kleunen JP, et al. The tension required at repair to re-appose the supraspinatus tendon to bone rapidly increases after injury. Clin Orthop Relat Res 2004;426:258–65.
37. Gimbel JA, Van Kleunen JP, Mehta S, et al. Supraspinatus tendon organizational and mechanical properties in a chronic rotator cuff tear animal model. J Biomech 2004;37(5):739–49.
38. Coleman SH, Fealy S, Ehteshami JR, et al. Chronic rotator cuff injury and repair model in sheep. J Bone Joint Surg Am 2003;85-A(12):2391–402.
39. Bassett RW, Cofield RH. Acute tears of the rotator cuff. The timing of surgical repair. Clin Orthop Relat Res 1983;175:18–24.
40. Bedi A, Dines J, Warren RF, et al. Massive tears of the rotator cuff. J Bone Joint Surg Am 2010;92(9):1894–908.
41. Clement ND, Hallett A, MacDonald D, et al. Does diabetes affect outcome after arthroscopic repair of the rotator cuff? J Bone Joint Surg Br 2010;92(8):1112–7.
42. Sherman SL, Lyman S, Koulouvaris P, et al. Risk factors for readmission and revision surgery following rotator cuff repair. Clin Orthop Relat Res 2008;466(3):608–13.

43. Galatz LM, Silva MJ, Rothermich SY, et al. Nicotine delays tendon-to-bone heal-
    ing in a rat shoulder model. J Bone Joint Surg Am 2006;88(9):2027–34.
44. Mallon WJ, Misamore G, Snead DS, et al. The impact of preoperative smoking habits
    on the results of rotator cuff repair. J Shoulder Elbow Surg 2004;13(2):129–32.
45. Cummins CA, Murrell GA. Mode of failure for rotator cuff repair with suture
    anchors identified at revision surgery. J Shoulder Elbow Surg 2003;12(2):128–33.
46. Piasecki DP, Verma NN, Nho SJ, et al. Outcomes after arthroscopic revision
    rotator cuff repair. Am J Sports Med 2010;38(1):40–6.
47. Lo IK, Burkhart SS. Arthroscopic revision of failed rotator cuff repairs: technique
    and results. Arthroscopy 2004;20(3):250–67.
48. Djurasovic M, Marra G, Arroyo JS, et al. Revision rotator cuff repair: factors influ-
    encing results. J Bone Joint Surg Am 2001;83-A(12):1849–55.
49. Neviaser RJ. Evaluation and management of failed rotator cuff repairs. Orthop
    Clin North Am 1997;28(2):215–24.
50. Sonnabend DH, Howlett CR, Young AA. Histological evaluation of repair of the
    rotator cuff in a primate model. J Bone Joint Surg Br 2010;92(4):586–94.
51. Athwal GS, Sperling JW, Rispoli DM, et al. Deep infection after rotator cuff repair.
    J Shoulder Elbow Surg 2007;16(3):306–11.
52. Herrera MF, Bauer G, Reynolds F, et al. Infection after mini-open rotator cuff
    repair. J Shoulder Elbow Surg 2002;11(6):605–8.
53. Castoldi F, Blonna D, Hertel R. External rotation lag sign revisited: accuracy for
    diagnosis of full thickness supraspinatus tear. J Shoulder Elbow Surg 2009;
    18(4):529–34.
54. Walch G, Boulahia A, Calderone S, et al. The 'dropping' and 'hornblower's' signs
    in evaluation of rotator-cuff tears. J Bone Joint Surg Br 1998;80(4):624–8.
55. Burkhart SS, Tehrany AM. Arthroscopic subscapularis tendon repair: technique
    and preliminary results. Arthroscopy 2002;18(5):454–63.
56. Motamedi AR, Urrea LH, Hancock RE, et al. Accuracy of magnetic resonance
    imaging in determining the presence and size of recurrent rotator cuff tears.
    J Shoulder Elbow Surg 2002;11(1):6–10.
57. Burkhart SS, Barth JR, Richards DP, et al. Arthroscopic repair of massive rotator cuff
    tears with stage 3 and 4 fatty degeneration. Arthroscopy 2007;23(4):347–54.
58. Prickett WD, Teefey SA, Galatz LM, et al. Accuracy of ultrasound imaging of the
    rotator cuff in shoulders that are painful postoperatively. J Bone Joint Surg Am
    2003;85-A(6):1084–9.
59. Bigliani LU, Cordasco FA, McIlveen SJ, et al. Operative treatment of failed repairs
    of the rotator cuff. J Bone Joint Surg Am 1992;74(10):1505–15.
60. DeOrio JK, Cofield RH. Results of a second attempt at surgical repair of a failed
    initial rotator-cuff repair. J Bone Joint Surg Am 1984;66(4):563–7.
61. Lädermann A, Denard PJ, Burkhart SS. Mid-term outcome of arthroscopic revi-
    sion repair of massive and nonmassive rotator cuff. Arthroscopy 2011;27(12):
    1620–7.
62. Levy O, Mullett H, Roberts S, et al. The role of anterior deltoid reeducation in
    patients with massive irreparable degenerative rotator cuff tears. J Shoulder
    Elbow Surg 2008;17(6):863–70.
63. Bell R. Arthroscopic repair of the rotator cuff. In: Edward VC, editor. Master
    techniques of orthopaedic surgery—the shoulder. Philadelphia: Lippincott;
    2004. p. 35–57.
64. Craig E. Techniques for full thickness rotator cuff repairs. In: Edward VC, editor.
    Master techniques in orthopaedic surgery—the shoulder. Philadelphia: Lippin-
    cott; 2004. p. 309–40.

65. Gamradt S, Rodeo S, Warren R. Platelet rich plasma in rotator cuff surgery. Tech Orthop 2007;22(1):26–33.
66. Warner JP, Krushell RJ, Masquelet A, et al. Anatomy and relationships of the suprascapular nerve: anatomical constraints to mobilization of the supraspinatus and infraspinatus muscles in the management of massive rotator-cuff tears. J Bone Joint Surg Am 1992;74(1):36–45.
67. Kovacevic D, Fox AJ, Bedi A, et al. Calcium-phosphate matrix with or without TGF-{beta}3 improves tendone-bone healing after rotator cuff repair. Am J Sports Med 2001;39:811–9.
68. Uggen C, Dines J, McGarry M, et al. The effect of recombinant human platelet derived growth factor BB-coated sutures on rotator cuff healing in a sheep model. Arthroscopy 2010;26(11):1456–62.
69. Ide J, Kikukawa K, Hirose J, et al. The effects of fibroblast growth factor-2 on rotator cuff reconstruction with acellular dermal matrix grafts. Arthroscopy 2009;25(6):608–16.
70. Gulotta LV, Kovacevic D, Packer JD, et al. Bone marrow-derived mesenchymal stem cells transduced with scleraxis improve rotator cuff healing in a rat model. Am J Sports Med 2011;39(6):1282–9.
71. Gulotta LV, Kovacevic D, Montgomery S, et al. Stem cells genetically modified with the developmental gene MT1-MMP improve regeneration of the supraspinatus tendon-to-bone insertion site. Am J Sports Med 2010;38(7):1429–37.
72. Randelli P, Arrigone P, Ragone V, et al. Platelet rich plasma in arthroscopic rotator cuff repair: a prospective RCT study, 2-year follow-up. J Shoulder Elbow Surg 2011;20:518–28.
73. Castricini R, Longo UG, Benedetto M, et al. Platelet-rich plasma augmentation for arthroscopic rotator cuff repair: a randomized controlled trial. Am J Sports Med 2011;39(2):258–65.
74. Rodeo SA, Delos D, Williams RJ III, et al. The effect of platelet-rich fibrin matrix on rotator cuff tendon healing: a prospective, randomized clinical study [abstract 9624]. In: Programs and abstracts of the American Orthopaedic Society for Sports Medicine Specialty Day Meeting. San Diego, July 7–10, 2011.

Revision Rotator Cuff Repair

Jay D. Keener, MD

KEYWORDS

- Rotator cuff • Revision • Failed rotator cuff

KEY POINTS

- Failure of tendon healing may or may not be the cause of persistent shoulder pain following rotator cuff repair, as errors in identifying the proper diagnosis can occur.
- Complete evaluation of the shoulder is needed to identify and treat potential confounding pain generators.
- If a recurrent tear is found to be repairable, the results of the surgery are encouraging, although persistent limitations in shoulder function are common. Strategies to improve the rates of tendon healing should be used and include the use of stronger repair constructs, when possible, and implementation of a slower rehabilitation progression.

Rotator cuff repair is one of the most common procedures performed in the shoulder. Predictable pain relief and functional improvements are seen across all age groups. However, anatomic healing of the surgically repaired tendon is not as consistent and has varied widely in the literature. In some patients, failure of tendon healing does not preclude a good clinical result.[1–3] However, several studies have directly correlated function and shoulder strength with healed repairs.[4–13] Failure of tendon healing is likely to be tolerated in younger patients or those who are engaged in activities that place higher demands on the shoulder. The goal of surgery, therefore, is ultimately to obtain healing after repair to maximize the chance of clinical success.

Failure of tendon healing may or may not be the cause of persistent shoulder pain following rotator cuff repair, as errors in identifying the proper diagnosis can occur. Failure of tendon healing is usually a result of the impaired biology of the damaged tendon or the intrinsic healing ability of the patient, as most contemporary tendon repair constructs possess adequate biomechanical strength to allow sufficient healing. However, the failure of healing is often multifactorial, and surgical technical errors or inappropriate rehabilitation may also affect tendon integrity. The biologic factors that most consistently correlate with failure of tendon healing are advanced patient age, larger tear size (>3 cm), and advanced muscle fatty degeneration.[4,5,9,14–18] These same factors also play a role in the likelihood of successful healing in the patient undergoing revision rotator cuff repair.

Shoulder and Elbow Service, Department of Orthopaedic Surgery, Washington University, Campus Box #8233, 660 South Euclid Avenue, St Louis, MO 63110, USA
E-mail address: keenerj@wudosis.wustl.edu

Clin Sports Med 31 (2012) 713–725
http://dx.doi.org/10.1016/j.csm.2012.07.007
0278-5919/12/$ – see front matter © 2012 Elsevier Inc. All rights reserved.

Consideration for attempted revision rotator cuff repair is appropriate in select cases when pain and limited shoulder function are seen in the context of a failed cuff repair. Appropriate indications are predicated on a thorough clinical examination and radiological workup of the patient to rule out associated potential causes of referred pain and concomitant diagnoses in the shoulder. These steps are necessary to ensure the formulation of a correct diagnosis and maximize the outcome of the patient.

The purpose of this article is to review the appropriate evaluation and management of patients with a failed rotator cuff repair, with specific emphasis on identifying proper surgical candidates for revision rotator cuff repair. This article also reviews the relevant surgical techniques, appropriate rehabilitation, and expected outcomes of revision rotator cuff repair surgery.

PATIENT EVALUATION

A complete evaluation of the patient with a failed rotator cuff repair surgery begins with a thorough history. Knowledge of the inciting events and duration of symptoms before the initial surgery is helpful to establish the chronicity of the tear and provide clues as to why the initial surgery failed. It is also helpful to review the postoperative rehabilitation course to ensure that the proper sequence of rehabilitation and timeline for progression of activities was followed. Progression of active range of motion and strengthening activities too quickly is probably an underrecognized cause of tendon failure. Although the true timeline for healing of cuff repairs in humans is not known, failure of the repair construct typically occurs within the first 3 months, a time when rapid progression of rehabilitation and activities can cause structural failure of the repair.[19]

When possible, review of prior operative notes can be helpful. Determining the quality of the torn tendon and type of repair construct used can clue the clinician to the potential success for healing of the initial surgery. Repairs performed under tension or tears repaired with nonanatomic repair constructs (margin convergence) likely signify more chronic tears with greater tendon retraction or tendon loss at the index procedure. Associated procedures such as biceps tenotomy or tenodesis, distal clavicle resection, or the presence of articular cartilage damage should be noted as well.

Patients should be questioned about their postoperative recovery course as well. It may be helpful to make a distinction between those patients who recovered well for several months, for example, and those who had persistent pain and/or difficulty in progression through the normal postoperative recovery milestones. In addition, care should be taken to review the job and recreational demands of the patients to better understand the expected physical demands to be placed on the injured shoulder.

The physical examination for the patient with a failed rotator cuff repair is similar to the examination of patients who have not had surgery, but should be expanded to look for other potential pain generators and possible causes of referred pain. Inspection should include assessment of atrophy within the supraspinatus and infraspinatus fossa. For open repairs, the deltoid should be assessed for local tenderness, atrophy, or signs of failure of healing to the acromion. Tenderness to palpation at the acromio-clavicular joint, the acromion, and the biceps groove should be elicited.

Active range of motion of the shoulder includes assessment of elevation with observation of scapular motion. Scapular substitution is a sign of cuff weakness or residual capsular stiffness. Scapular winging or dyskinesia should be evaluated with specific assessment of the strength of isolated scapular stabilizer muscle weakness when indicated. The presence of pseudoparalysis, or the inability to elevate the shoulder against gravity, usually indicates a massive cuff tear. In these patients, the deltoid and axillary nerve should also be carefully examined, as an unrecognized axillary nerve injury must be ruled out. Proximal humeral escape with attempted elevation is an onerous sign usually indicating a massive cuff tear combined with insufficiency of the anterior deltoid and/or anterior acromion, often iatrogenic in nature. Assessment of active range should also include external rotation with the arm at the side and with the shoulder abducted 90° in the plane of the scapula. The presence of external rotation lag signs usually signifies larger tears with involvement of the infraspinatus and possibly the teres minor. Painful internal rotation motion loss is common in patients with cuff disease and should be assessed in comparison to the opposite shoulder.

When deficits in active range of motion are seen, passive range of motion should be assessed to determine the available range of motion of the glenohumeral joint and capsuloligamentous structures. Limitation of passive motion, especially external rotation, is a sign of residual capsular stiffness or significant underlying glenohumeral joint arthritis. Strength testing of the rotator cuff muscles is performed in isolation to assess for strength and pain. Special tests to identify pain at the acromioclavicular joint and the biceps tendon should be performed as well. Pain radiating below the elbow or along the medial scapula indicates referred pain from the cervical spine. Cervical spine range of motion and the Spurlings maneuver can help identify concomitant cervical radiculopathy. A careful neurologic examination of the upper extremity should be performed when indicated.

RADIOLOGIC IMAGING

Routine shoulder radiographs are helpful after failed cuff repair surgery. The glenohumeral joint space should be evaluated for joint space narrowing and/or evidence of proximal humeral migration. Subtle migration may be more readily apparent by looking at asymmetry between the inferior and superior joint spaces rather than narrowing of the acromiohumeral interval. Advanced glenohumeral joint space narrowing and/or proximal migration in the setting of a failed cuff repair is a relative contraindication for attempted revision cuff repair surgery. The acromion should be evaluated, especially after open rotator cuff repair surgery to ensure that overaggressive acromial resection or anterior acromionectomy has not been performed. Assessment of the bone stock of the greater tuberosity is an important factor when considering revision cuff repair and may be influenced by previous cuff repair constructs.

Advanced soft tissue imaging is critical when evaluating patients with failure of healing after rotator cuff repair, because many of the decisions regarding future surgery are based on these studies. Magnetic resonance imaging (MRI) is the most commonly used modality in evaluating shoulder pain before surgery and can still be helpful after surgery; however, artifact from previous surgery, especially when metal anchors are used, can decrease the accuracy of the test. The addition of arthrogram dye is helpful for identifying recurrent full-thickness cuff tears and improved accuracy for identifying associated labral tears. MRI is most accurate for identifying recurrent full-thickness cuff defects and quantifying the degree of tendon retraction and cuff muscle fatty degeneration and atrophy, all of which are important factors to consider before revision surgery. Likewise, computed tomographic (CT) arthrogram can accurately identify a recurrent full-thickness cuff defect and stage the amount of muscle degenerative changes that have occurred. With both MRI and CT arthrogram, careful assessment of the pattern of muscle changes can better clue the clinician into the pattern and chronicity of the tendon tear. A previous double-row repair that has retorn may result in substantial tendon loss, because the rupture may occur at the medial row of anchors.[20,21] Special attention to the subscapularis and biceps tendons should be given, especially in the context of failed cuff repair, because unrecognized injuries to these tissues can be a source of persistent pain and should be addressed. Advanced imaging can also identify the presence of associated pathologies, such as an os acromiale, spinoglenoid cysts, and isolated articular cartilage defects, which may affect the treatment of these patients.

Shoulder ultrasonography is a useful modality in evaluating patients with recurrent cuff defects, because this test is less susceptible to metal and suture artifact from previous surgery. Furthermore, shoulder ultrasonography is a dynamic study, which, theoretically, can better differentiate recurrent cuff defects from subacromial scarring, which may be mistaken for a healed tendon on MRI. Shoulder ultrasound has been studied in the postoperative shoulder compared with arthroscopic findings, demonstrating a sensitivity of 91%, specificity of 86%, and overall accuracy of 89% for the detection of full-thickness recurrent cuff tears.[22] One major drawback regarding ultrasonography is the learning curve associated with this test and its limited availability. However, in recent years, more orthopaedic surgeons have been using this modality with reasonable accuracy.

In recent years, more attention has been given to the suprascapular nerve as a cause of pain and weakness in patients with rotator cuff tears. In larger, more retracted tears, there is a theoretic tensioning or kinking of the nerve at the level of the suprascapular or spinoglenoid notch with tendon retraction. One study demonstrated signs of supraspinatus and/or infraspinatus muscle denervation in 38% of massive cuff tears.[23] The author believes that electromyography should be considered in recurrent cuff tears in which weakness in external rotation or atrophy of the infraspinatus is greater than expected, given the size of the cuff tear and in cases where neurogenic edema is seen within the supraspinatus or infraspinatus muscle bellies.

SURGICAL INDICATIONS/CONTRAINDICATIONS

The indications for revision cuff repair are similar to those of primary repair: pain and limited function in the setting of a recurrent cuff tear. However, specific tear and patient-related factors must be carefully considered in the revision setting. Furthermore, realistic patient expectations must be carefully reviewed with the patient, because the results of revision surgery are less predictable than primary surgery both in terms of clinical outcomes and expectations for tendon healing. Ultimately, the ability to repair the tendon defect adequately cannot be fully determined until the time of surgery. To optimize outcomes, the passive range of motion and flexibility of the shoulder should be optimized before surgery. When necessary, glenohumeral injections and physical therapy should be used to restore mobility to the joint, because a stiff shoulder before surgery is sure to be even stiffer after surgery.

Attempted revision cuff repair is ideally indicated for recurrent tears in motivated patients with a reasonable chance for tendon healing. Ideally, patients should be less than 60 to 65 years of age, the deltoid muscle should be healthy, overhead elevation should be greater than 90°, the muscles of the torn tendons should not have advanced fatty degeneration (Goutallier grade 2 or less), and reasonable tendon quality should be present on advanced imaging. Revision repair is attempted in cases when more advanced muscle changes or tendon retractions are seen in smaller recurrent tears, but these are not ideal circumstances. In situations with advanced muscle atrophy and poorer tendon quality, a partial tendon repair is considered, because this may help to restore the rotator cuff force couple and improve shoulder function.[24–26] However, there are limited outcomes data for partial repairs performed in the revision setting. In cases with deltoid injury, attempted revision cuff repair is performed open through the deltoid defect with meticulous repair of the deltoid back to the acromion. The use of biologic augmentation of the deltoid may help augment deltoid repair in cases of poorer tissue quality.[27]

In cases of complete supraspinatus and infraspinatus tears with advanced muscle and/or tendon changes, the subscapularis and deltoid are intact, and there is minimal glenohumeral arthritis, and latissimus dorsi tendon transfer should be entertained. This surgery is more reliable for pain relief and for restoring external rotation motion than for improving elevation motion, although some improvement in elevation is sometimes noted.[28-31] These patients should be highly motivated as the duration of recovery is long. In addition, tendon transfers are probably less reliable for restoring durable function in manual laborers. For older patients, greater than 60 to 65 years of age, with pain, limited active elevation, and glenohumeral arthritis, reverse total shoulder arthroplasty is a more reliable procedure.

Active infection, axillary nerve injury, and proximal humeral escape are absolute contraindications for revision cuff repair. Revision cuff repair should not be performed when 2 or more tendons are torn and advanced atrophy or fatty changes are seen in the involved muscles, unless a partial repair is thought to be a possibility. Many of these patients will have significant proximal humeral migration and early arthritic changes in the glenohumeral joint on plain radiographs. Advanced age, greater than 65 years, and pseudoparalysis of the shoulder are relative contraindications for surgery. In addition, iatrogenic severe deltoid injury or anterior acromial resection or insufficiency often results in pseudoparalysis, proximal humeral escape, and/or limited elevation motion. In these patients, the outcomes of revision cuff repair are less predictable. Severe bone loss of the greater tuberosity from previous anchor placement or bone tunnels may compromise fixation of the repair and should be carefully assessed before revision surgery. A symptomatic os acromiale is also a relative contraindication for revision cuff repair.

SURGICAL TECHNIQUE

Before surgery, a complete assessment of all potential pain generators within the shoulder is performed to develop a surgical strategy. The decision to perform a distal clavicle resection or release of the suprascapular nerve, for instance, is made before surgery based on the physical examination and diagnostic studies.

The author prefers to perform a revision cuff repair in the beach chair position using arm holders that allow inferior traction to the shoulder to improve visualization in the subacromial space, although lateral decubitus positioning can be used based on surgeon preference. The procedure is preferred to be performed arthroscopically; however, a mini-open approach can be used and is indicated in cases where deltoid repair or bone tunnels are needed. The surgery begins with a thorough diagnostic arthroscopy with assessment of the biceps tendon, glenoid labrum, glenoid and humeral head articular cartilage, and the rotator cuff tendons, including the subscapularis. A biceps procedure is indicated in cases where preoperative biceps findings are positive, when biceps degeneration or instability is seen, or, less commonly, when a superior labral tear is noted. The decision to perform a biceps tenodesis or tenotomy is based on the preference of the surgeon and is generally influenced by the age, body habitus, and physical demands of the patient. Instability of the biceps tendon implies disruption of the medial biceps sling and is sometimes associated with upper subscapularis tendon tears, which must be carefully evaluated. Consideration for biceps tenotomy or tenodesis should be entertained when a recurrent tear of the anterior supraspinatus tendon is seen. In these cases, entrapment of the biceps tendon may occur after repair, and avoiding late onset biceps symptoms is preferable.

The subacromial space is inspected to identify the recurrent tear and assess tendon quality and mobility. Previous suture material should be removed. When possible, previous anchors within the apex of the greater tuberosity are removed, especially when there is a potential for crowding of anchors or in cases with limited bone stock of the tuberosity. The torn tendons must be separated from surrounding adhesions, which are common between the tendon and the deltoid fascia and the surrounding bursa. Tendon retraction can be severe. Complete glenoid and bursal side releases are performed to improve mobility. Releases are facilitated by placing traction sutures through the retracted tendon edge. On the deep side of the tendon, the capsule is released with care taken posteriorly not to damage the suprascapular nerve in the spinoglenoid notch, which lies 15 to 20 mm posterior to the glenoid edge.[32] For retracted supraspinatus tears, all soft tissue attachments anteriorly between the supraspinatus and the coracoid (coracohumeral ligaments) and glenoid are released (**Fig. 1**). An anterior interval slide is performed, releasing the front edge of the supraspinatus tendon from the interval capsule. Subacromial releases are generally complete posteriorly when the spine of the scapula is visible. Once full releases are performed, the tear pattern is assessed as well as the mobility of the tendon to determine if the tendon can reach the greater tuberosity without undo tension.

Anatomic repairs require adequate tendon mobility to reach and cover the tuberosity. Before anchor placement, the greater tuberosity is roughened with a shaver or burr to create a bleeding bed. When tendon mobility is good, the author prefers to secure the tendon with a double-row transosseous repair construct (**Fig. 2**). Although double-row repairs are biomechanically stronger and restore the native footprint anatomy better than single-row repairs,[33–39] the potential benefits for tendon

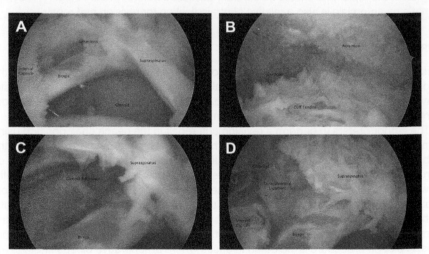

Fig. 1. (*A*) Recurrent supraspinatus tear of the left shoulder as viewed from a lateral subacromial portal. Severe retraction of the anterior supraspinatus is seen with a split between the anterior supraspinatus and the interval capsule. Adhesion between the tendon edge and biceps anchor are noted. (*B*) Left shoulder. Soft tissue adhesions between the supraspinatus and the acromion have been released. The superficial coracohumeral ligament attachments from the coracoid base to the supraspinatus have been divided. (*C*) Left shoulder. Adhesions between the undersurface of the supraspinatus tendon and the glenoid and biceps anchor are released. (*D*) Left shoulder. An anterior interval slide is performed releasing the interval capsule from the anterior supraspinatus. The deep coracohumeral ligaments are divided freeing the anterior supraspinatus completely.

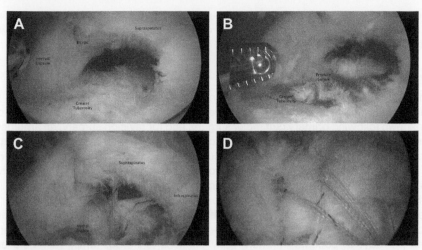

Fig. 2. (*A*) Small recurrent left shoulder supraspinatus tear as viewed from a lateral subacromial portal. Moderate tendon retraction is seen with minimal tendon loss. The anchor sutures from the previous single row repair are seen in the greater tuberosity. (*B*) Left shoulder. The greater tuberosity is cleared of soft tissue and lightly decorticated to facilitate a healthy bleeding bone surface. (*C*) Left shoulder. A medial-row anchor has been placed just lateral to the articular margin, and the medial-row sutures have been passed through the torn tendon with care taken not to trap the biceps tendon. (*D*) Left shoulder. Double-row repair of the recurrent cuff tendon viewed from a lateral subacromial portal.

healing are debatable, and the clinical outcomes of these repairs have not been shown to be greater than single-row repairs.[40–45] However, these repair constructs have not been compared in the revision setting, and the theoretical benefit of a double-row repair may be justified in the revision setting. These constructs may be especially relevant in a shoulder that has failed to heal with previous simpler repair constructs.

For tears with greater retraction than sagittal plane width and/or tears with limited mobility, nonanatomic repair techniques such as margin convergence sutures are performed. Margin convergence effectively lateralizes the torn tendon edge, allowing coverage of the humeral head and closure of the defect.

The tendon edge is then repaired to the tuberosity with suture anchors either with a single-row construct or a double-row construct if the tendon edge will cover most of the tuberosity. In cases with tendon loss, the tendon can be repaired in a more medial position on the greater tuberosity with suture anchors; the author prefers triple-loaded anchors to achieve more points of fixation within the tendon. In some instances, only a partial tendon repair is possible. If the infraspinatus can be repaired to the tuberosity, the rotator cuff force couple can, theoretically, be reestablished, which may allow pain relief and restoration of shoulder function.

The use of biologic augmentation may play a role in revision tendon repair when tendon quality is poor or a persistent defect in the tendon is noted. The most popular graft choices currently used are composed of allograft tissue. The use of xenografts has been associated with high failure rates and potential complications. There are limited unbiased data regarding the results of tendon graft augmentation, especially in a revision repair setting. The author prefers to use grafts to augment a repairable tendon (rather than span a tendon defect) with poor tissue quality in a younger patient. In shoulders with defect that is not repairable, a partial repair or possible latissimus dorsi transfer is preferred than a graft augmentation. The placement of these grafts is performed open or arthroscopically, depending on surgeon experience. The potential indications for graft augmentation are controversial, and refined indications will likely be seen in the future.

POSTOPERATIVE REHABILITATION

Preference for a conservative progression of rehabilitation milestones is given to patients undergoing a revision rotator cuff repair. The optimal period of immobilization is unknown following primary cuff repair surgery, and for revision surgery, an argument is made to progress rehabilitation milestones more slowly to allow for adequate tendon healing. The timeline for mature cuff repair healing in humans is unknown, but it is generally believed to occur at 3 to 4 months. Most cases of postoperative repair failure are believed to occur in the first 3 to 6 months after surgery.

The author prefers to immobilize the shoulder in a sling and abduction pillow for 6 weeks after revision rotator cuff repair. Patients are permitted to remove the sling periodically for range of motion activities of the elbow, forearm, wrist, and hand several times per day. In patients in whom early stiffness is noted, family members are instructed in passive external rotation stretching with the arm at the side. At 6 weeks, passive range of motion in physical therapy in initiated; however, true active assistive and active range of motion exercises are avoided until 3 months after surgery. At this point, active assistive and active motion is initiated in the form of pulley exercises, supine elevation, and other exercises as directed by the therapist. Internal rotation stretching, especially behind the back should be avoided until 3 months after surgery, because these positions stretch the repair maximally. Care is taken to facilitate proper scapular mechanics with active range of motion before initiating rotator cuff strengthening exercises. Rotator cuff, deltoid, and scapular stabilizer strengthening exercises are generally initiated at 4 months after surgery, if good progression has been seen with previous activities. Strengthening and conditioning are continued with home exercises up to 6 months after surgery.

OUTCOMES

There are several studies reporting the results of open and, more recently, arthroscopic revision rotator cuff repair surgery. The clinical results of revision rotator cuff repair are not as successful or as predictable as primary cuff surgery; however, the outcomes are improved in most cases. The difficulty in applying the results of these studies to clinical practice lies in patient selection, as the ability to repair a recurrent tear is sometimes unknown until the time of surgery. Furthermore, no presurgical tests are definitive in predicting whether or not the tear is repairable. Therefore, preoperative patient counseling must be tempered somewhat in case an irreparable defect is encountered at the time of surgery.

REVISION OPEN REPAIRS

The initial results of revision surgery pertained to open surgery. DeOrio and Cofield[46] initially reported sobering results. In a group of revision cuff repairs, although 76% of patients had substantial pain relief, 63% still had moderate to severe pain. Functional gains in this group were minimal, with a mean abduction increase of 8°. Overall, 58% were considered to have a poor outcome. In Harryman and colleagues'[9] classic paper regarding the results of open cuff repairs, 18 of the 105 shoulders had a revision surgery. Of these 18, 10 were repairs isolated to the supraspinatus tendon; 3 were supraspinatus and infraspinatus tears; and 5 involved the supraspinatus, infraspinatus, and the subscapularis. Healing of the repairs was noted in 8 of the 18 shoulders. In those shoulders with healed repairs, the clinical outcomes were similar to healed repairs after primary surgery.

Bigliani and colleagues[47] in 1992 reported the results of 31 revision open rotator cuff repairs. The mean age of the cohort was 57 years, and there were 12 massive, 10 large, 7 medium, and 1 small tears noted at surgery. Using a modified Neer score, only 52% had a satisfactory clinical result; however, 81% had good to excellent pain relief following surgery. The mean elevation motion improved from 76° to 112°, and the mean external rotation motion improved approximately 20°. The author believed that poor-quality tissue and deltoid insufficiency were related to poorer results after revision surgery and that inadequate repair, deltoid insufficiency, and persistent acromial impingement were related to failure of the index surgery. Neviaser and colleagues[48] reported the clinical results of 50 revision open rotator cuff repairs, noting 90% patient satisfaction with a mean of 30-months follow-up. Pain relief was noted in 92% of patients; however, improvement of function was less consistent as just more than half the patients had improvement in elevation motion. Djurasovic and colleagues,[49] in the largest series of revision rotator cuff repairs reviewed the results of 80 revision open cuff repairs. The mean age of the patients was 59 years, and the mean duration of follow-up was 49 months. Overall, 69% of patients had a satisfactory result according to the modified Neer score. The mean Visual Analogue Scale (VAS) pain score improved from 7.4 to 3.0, the mean active elevation improved from 105 to 140, and mean external rotation improved from 39° to 54°. Tears were subdivided into large/massive and small/medium size for comparison. Tear size at the time of revision did not affect outcome; however, tears that were small or medium in size at the index surgery had better results after revision surgery. Factors that influenced outcomes included preoperative elevation greater than 90°, an intact deltoid, good-quality rotator cuff tissue, and only one previous attempted rotator cuff repair. All patients who met these criteria had a satisfactory result.

REVISION ARTHROSCOPIC REPAIRS

In recent years, the results of arthroscopic revision cuff repairs have been reported as well. The first series reported by Lo and colleagues,[50] in 2004, examined the outcomes of 14 patients with a mean age of 58 years treated after revision arthroscopic repair. Eleven massive-sized, one large-sized, and 2 medium-sized tears were noted. At a mean of 24 months, 13 of the 14 patients were satisfied with the procedure. The mean Univeristy of California Los Angeles (UCLA) score increased from 13 points preoperatively to 29 points following surgery, and there were 9 good/excellent and 5 fair/poor results. The mean elevation improved from 121° to 154°, and the mean external rotation motion improved from 26° to 44°.

Keener and Colleagues[51] reported the results of 21 patients after revision arthroscopic rotator cuff repair with both clinical outcomes and healing data. The mean age of the patient was 56 years, and 10 recurrent tears involved a single tendon, whereas 11 tears involved more than one tendon. Eighteen of 21 repairs were performed with a double-row technique. At a mean of 33 months, significant improvements were seen in VAS pain score, Simple Shoulder Test (SST) score, American Shoulder and Elbow Surgeons (ASES) score, active elevation, and external rotation motion. Overall, tendon healing was noted in 48% of shoulders, with 70% healing in single tendon compared with 27% healing in multitendon repairs (statistically significant). Tendon healing had no effect on outcomes measures with the exception of the Constant score, which was higher in shoulders with intact tendons. The average age of patients (52 years) with healed tendons was significantly less than those with recurrent tears (59 years).

Piasecki and colleagues[52] gave a retrospective review of 54 patients, 72% of which were worker's compensation claims, following arthroscopic revision rotator cuff repair. The mean age of the patients was 55 years, and the mean duration of follow-up was 31 months. There were 33 (61%) single-tendon tears and 21 (39%) multitendon tears. Sixty-one percent of the tears were repaired with a double-row technique. Significant improvements were noted in the mean VAS pain score (decreased from 5.2–2.8), SST (increased from 3.6–7.5), ASES score (increased from 44–68) and elevation range of motion (increased from 121–136). Six patients (11%) failed and required further surgery. The major risk factor for need for repeat revision was a history of more than one previous surgery. Clinical failures, also defined as a postoperative ASES score of 50 points or less, was more common in female patients and those with preoperative elevation less than 120° and preoperative abduction of less than 90°. Tear size at the time of surgery did not affect clinical results and the author did not assess for tendon healing after surgery.

One recent study reported the results of 72 revision arthroscopic rotator cuff repairs, including 53 massive tears.[53] The mean age of the patients was 60 years, and the mean follow-up period was 63 months. Surgeries included complete and partial repairs with a variety of techniques including margin convergence repair as well as single-row and double-row repairs. Overall, 78% of patients were satisfied with the result. Significant improvements were seen in pain, range of motion, and shoulder function with no difference between massive and small tears. With the nonmassive tears, the mean UCLA score improved from 18 to 26 with 52% good and excellent results compared with an improvement from 17 to 26 with 50% good and excellent results in the massive group. Repeat surgery was needed in close to 10% of the subjects. In this study, female gender, modest limitation of forward elevation, and a preoperative VAS pain score of greater than 5 correlated with a poorer clinical result.

Looking at the outcomes data as a whole, several observations can be seen. Revision cuff repair is more reliable for pain relief than restoration of function. Most patients reported in these series are relatively young with mean ages in the mid-50s. The size of the recurrent tear does not appear to effect clinical outcomes, although inadequate power may be a factor in many of these studies. More than one previous attempted repair, poor-quality tissue and a lack of overhead motion before surgery are risk factors for clinical failure of revision cuff repair surgery.

SUMMARY

The management of patients with a failed rotator cuff repair is challenging. Revision arthroscopic repairs can be entertained in select patients when realistic outcomes are understood. Complete evaluation of the shoulder is needed to identify and treat potential confounding pain generators. The ability to determine if a recurrent tear is repairable is difficult, because there are no established criteria to make this determination. If a recurrent tear is found to be repairable, the results of the surgery are encouraging, although persistent limitations in shoulder function are common. Strategies to improve the rates of tendon healing should be used and include the use of stronger repair constructs, when possible, and implementation of a slower rehabilitation progression.

REFERENCES

1. Galatz LM, Ball CM, Teefey SA, et al. The outcome and repair integrity of completely arthroscopically repaired large and massive rotator cuff tears. J Bone Joint Surg Am 2004;86(2):219–24.

2. Ellman H, Kay SP, Wirth M. Arthroscopic treatment of full-thickness rotator cuff tears: 2- to 7-year follow-up study. Arthroscopy 1993;9(2):195–200.
3. Jost B, Pfirrmann CW, Gerber C, et al. Clinical outcome after structural failure of rotator cuff repairs. J Bone Joint Surg Am 2000;82(3):304–14.
4. Bishop J, Klepps S, Lo IK, et al. Cuff integrity after arthroscopic versus open rotator cuff repair: a prospective study. J Shoulder Elbow Surg 2006;15(3):290–9.
5. Boileau P, Brassart N, Watkinson DJ, et al. Arthroscopic repair of full-thickness tears of the supraspinatus: does the tendon really heal? J Bone Joint Surg Am 2005;87(6):1229–40.
6. DeFranco MJ, Bershadsky B, Ciccone J, et al. Functional outcome of arthroscopic rotator cuff repairs: a correlation of anatomic and clinical results. J Shoulder Elbow Surg 2007;16(6):759–65.
7. Charousset C, Grimberg J, Duranthon LD, et al. The time for functional recovery after arthroscopic rotator cuff repair: correlation with tendon healing controlled by computed tomography arthrography. Arthroscopy 2008;24(1):25–33.
8. Anderson K, Boothby M, Aschenbrener D, et al. Outcome and structural integrity after arthroscopic rotator cuff repair using 2 rows of fixation: minimum 2-year follow-up. Am J Sports Med 2006;34(12):1899–905.
9. Harryman DT, Mack LA, Wang KY, et al. Repairs of the rotator cuff. Correlation of functional results with integrity of the cuff. J Bone Joint Surg Am 1991;73(7): 982–9.
10. Huijsmans PE, Pritchard MP, Berghs BM, et al. Arthroscopic rotator cuff repair with double-row fixation. J Bone Joint Surg Am 2007;89(6):1248–57.
11. Lafosse L, Brozska R, Toussaint B, et al. The outcome and structural integrity of arthroscopic rotator cuff repair with use of the double-row suture anchor technique. J Bone Joint Surg Am 2007;89(7):1533–41.
12. Levy O, Loeb M, Chuinard C, et al. Mid-term clinical and sonographic outcome of arthroscopic repair of the rotator cuff. J Bone Joint Surg Br 2008;90(10):1341–7.
13. Cole BJ, McCarty LP, Kang RW, et al. Arthroscopic rotator cuff repair: prospective functional outcome and repair integrity at minimum 2-year follow-up. J Shoulder Elbow Surg 2007;16(5):579–85.
14. Tashjian RZ, Hollins AM, Kim HM, et al. Factors affecting healing rates after arthroscopic double-row rotator cuff repair. Am J Sports Med 2010;38(12): 2435–42.
15. Kamath G, Galatz LM, Keener JD, et al. Tendon integrity and functional outcome after arthroscopic repair of high-grade partial-thickness supraspinatus tears. J Bone Joint Surg Am 2009;91(5):1055–62.
16. Gulotta LV, Nho SJ, Dodson CC, et al. Prospective evaluation of arthroscopic rotator cuff repairs at 5 years: part II–prognostic factors for clinical and radiographic outcomes. J Shoulder Elbow Surg 2011;20(6):941–6.
17. Sethi PM, Noonan BC, Cunningham J, et al. Repair results of 2-tendon rotator cuff tears utilizing the transosseous equivalent technique. J Shoulder Elbow Surg 2010;19(8):1210–7.
18. Nho SJ, Shindle MK, Adler RS, et al. Prospective analysis of arthroscopic rotator cuff repair: subgroup analysis. J Shoulder Elbow Surg 2009;18(5):697–704.
19. Miller BS, Downie BK, Kohen RB, et al. When do rotator cuff repairs fail? serial ultrasound examination after arthroscopic repair of large and massive rotator cuff tears. Am J Sports Med 2011;39(10):2064–70.
20. Hayashida K, Tanaka M, Koizumi K, et al. Characteristic retear patterns assessed by magnetic resonance imaging after arthroscopic double-row rotator cuff repair. Arthroscopy 2012;28(4):458–64.

21. Cho NS, Yi JW, Lee BG, et al. Retear patterns after arthroscopic rotator cuff repair: single-row versus suture bridge technique. Am J Sports Med 2010; 38(4):664–71.

22. Prickett WD, Teefey SA, Galatz LM, et al. Accuracy of ultrasound imaging of the rotator cuff in shoulders that are painful postoperatively. J Bone Joint Surg Am 2003;85-A(6):1084–9.

23. Costouros JG, Porramatikul M, Lie DT, et al. Reversal of suprascapular neuropathy following arthroscopic repair of massive supraspinatus and infraspinatus rotator cuff tears. Arthroscopy 2007;23(11):1152–61.

24. Iagulli ND, Field LD, Hobgood ER, et al. Comparison of partial versus complete arthroscopic repair of massive rotator cuff tears. Am J Sports Med 2012;40(5): 1022–6.

25. Kim SJ, Lee IS, Kim SH, et al. Arthroscopic partial repair of irreparable large to massive rotator cuff tears. Arthroscopy 2012;28(6):761–8.

26. Burkhart SS, Nottage WM, Ogilvie-Harris DJ, et al. Partial repair of irreparable rotator cuff tears. Arthroscopy 1994;10(4):363–70.

27. Chebli CM, Murthi AM. Deltoidplasty: outcomes using orthobiologic augmentation. J Shoulder Elbow Surg 2007;16(4):425–8.

28. Gerhardt C, Lehmann L, Lichtenberg S, et al. Modified L'Episcopo tendon transfers for irreparable rotator cuff tears: 5-year follow-up. Clin Orthop Relat Res 2010;468(6):1572–7.

29. Birmingham PM, Neviaser RJ. Outcome of latissimus dorsi transfer as a salvage procedure for failed rotator cuff repair with loss of elevation. J Shoulder Elbow Surg 2008;17(6):871–4.

30. Iannotti JP, Hennigan S, Herzog R, et al. Latissimus dorsi tendon transfer for irreparable posterosuperior rotator cuff tears. Factors affecting outcome. J Bone Joint Surg Am 2006;88(2):342–8.

31. Gerber C, Maquieira G, Espinosa N. Latissimus dorsi transfer for the treatment of irreparable rotator cuff tears. J Bone Joint Surg Am 2006;88(1):113–20.

32. Bigliani LU, Dalsey RM, McCann PD, et al. An anatomical study of the suprascapular nerve. Arthroscopy 1990;6(4):301–5.

33. Smith CD, Alexander S, Hill AM, et al. A biomechanical comparison of single and double-row fixation in arthroscopic rotator cuff repair. J Bone Joint Surg Am 2006; 88(11):2425–31.

34. Milano G, Grasso A, Zarelli D, et al. Comparison between single-row and double-row rotator cuff repair: a biomechanical study. Knee Surg Sports Traumatol Arthrosc 2008;16(1):75–80.

35. Meier SW, Meier JD. The effect of double-row fixation on initial repair strength in rotator cuff repair: a biomechanical study. Arthroscopy 2006;22(11):1168–73.

36. Ma CB, Comerford L, Wilson J, et al. Biomechanical evaluation of arthroscopic rotator cuff repairs: double-row compared with single-row fixation. J Bone Joint Surg Am 2006;88(2):403–10.

37. Kim DH, Elattrache NS, Tibone JE, et al. Biomechanical comparison of a single-row versus double-row suture anchor technique for rotator cuff repair. Am J Sports Med 2006;34(3):407–14.

38. Lorbach O, Bachelier F, Vees J, et al. Cyclic loading of rotator cuff reconstructions: single-row repair with modified suture configurations versus double-row repair. Am J Sports Med 2008;36(8):1504–10.

39. Ahmad CS, Kleweno C, Jacir AM, et al. Biomechanical performance of rotator cuff repairs with humeral rotation: a new rotator cuff repair failure model. Am J Sports Med 2008;36(5):888–92.

40. Sugaya H, Maeda K, Matsuki K, et al. Functional and structural outcome after arthroscopic full-thickness rotator cuff repair: single-row versus dual-row fixation. Arthroscopy 2005;21(11):1307–16.
41. Charousset C, Grimberg J, Duranthon LD, et al. Can a double-row anchorage technique improve tendon healing in arthroscopic rotator cuff repair?: A prospective, nonrandomized, comparative study of double-row and single-row anchorage techniques with computed tomographic arthrography tendon healing assessment. Am J Sports Med 2007;35(8):1247–53.
42. Franceschi F, Ruzzini L, Longo UG, et al. Equivalent clinical results of arthroscopic single-row and double-row suture anchor repair for rotator cuff tears: a randomized controlled trial. Am J Sports Med 2007;35(8):1254–60.
43. Burks RT, Crim J, Brown N, et al. A prospective randomized clinical trial comparing arthroscopic single- and double-row rotator cuff repair: magnetic resonance imaging and early clinical evaluation. Am J Sports Med 2009;37(4): 674–82.
44. Grasso A, Milano G, Salavatore M, et al. Single-row versus double-row arthroscopic rotator cuff repair: a prospective randomized clinical study. Arthroscopy 2009;25(1):4–12.
45. Koh KH, Kang KC, Lim TK, et al. Prospective randomized clinical trial of single-versus double-row suture anchor repair in 2- to 4-cm rotator cuff tears: clinical and magnetic resonance imaging results. Arthroscopy 2011;27(4):453–62.
46. DeOrio JK, Cofield RH. Results of a second attempt at surgical repair of a failed initial rotator-cuff repair. J Bone Joint Surg Am 1984;66(4):563–7.
47. Bigliani LU, Cordasco FA, McIlveen SJ, et al. Operative treatment of failed repairs of the rotator cuff. J Bone Joint Surg Am 1992;74(10):1505–15.
48. Neviaser RJ, Neviaser TJ. Operation for failed rotator cuff repair. Analysis of fifty cases. J Shoulder Elbow Surg 1992;1:283–6.
49. Djurasovic M, Marra G, Arroyo JS, et al. Revision rotator cuff repair: factors influencing results. J Bone Joint Surg Am 2001;83-A(12):1849–55.
50. Lo IK, Burkhart SS. Arthroscopic revision of failed rotator cuff repairs: technique and results. J Arthroscopy 2004;20(3):250–67.
51. Keener JD, Wei As, Kim HM, et al. Revision arthroscopic rotator cuff repair: repair integrity and clinical outcome. J Bone Joint Surg 2012;92(3):590–8.
52. Piasecki DP, Verma NN, Nho SJ, et al. Outcomes after arthroscopic revision rotator cuff repair. Am J Sports Med 2010;38(1):40–6.
53. Ladermann A, Denard PJ, Burkhart SS. Midterm outcome of arthroscopic revision repair of massive and nonmassive rotator cuff tears. Arthroscopy 2011;27(12): 1620–7.

Nonarthroplasty Options for the Management of Massive and Irreparable Rotator Cuff Tears

Ruth A. Delaney, MB BCh, BAO, MRCS[a], Albert Lin, MD[b],
Jon J.P. Warner, MD[c],*

KEYWORDS

- Massive rotator cuff tears • Subacromial decompression • Margin convergence
- Suprascapular nerve • Tendon transfers

KEY POINTS

- A massive rotator cuff tear is not necessarily irreparable, and an irreparable tear is not always massive. Number of tendons involved, tissue quality, and decreased acromiohumeral distance are as important as tear size in determining reparability.
- Debridement of irreparable tears may have a role in low functional demand patients but results deteriorate over time.
- Patients who do not have pseudoparalysis or advanced cuff tear arthropathy can benefit from biceps tenotomy or tenodesis.
- Suprascapular neuropathy has been shown to be a potential neurogenic cause of pain in massive rotator cuff tears.
- Tendon transfers offer good results in patients with massive, irreparable rotator cuff tears who have intact deltoid function and disabling weakness but not pseudoparalysis.

INTRODUCTION

The definition of massive or irreparable rotator cuff tears is not always consistent, but attempts have been made to rationalize this description. Patte[1] proposed a classification system of rotator cuff tears to allow comparison of treatment results for specific lesions and to allow analysis of results obtained by different groups and treatment regimens. He categorized tears based on the extent of the tear, the topography of the tear

Disclosures: The authors have identified no financial affiliations relevant to the topic of this article.
[a] Harvard Combined Orthopaedic Residency Program, Massachusetts General Hospital, WHT 535, Boston, MA 02114, USA; [b] Harvard Shoulder Service, Massachusetts General Hospital, Yawkey Suite 3G, Boston, MA 02114, USA; [c] Harvard Shoulder Service; Harvard Medical School, Massachusetts General Hospital, Yawkey Suite 3G, Boston, MA 02114, USA
* Corresponding author.
E-mail address: jwarner@partners.org

Clin Sports Med 31 (2012) 727–748
http://dx.doi.org/10.1016/j.csm.2012.07.008
0278-5919/12/$ – see front matter © 2012 Elsevier Inc. All rights reserved.

in the sagittal plane, the topography of the tear in the frontal plane, the quality of the muscle, and the state of the long head of the biceps. In terms of the extent of the tear, there were 4 groups of tear, with group III being large or massive tears defined as full substance tears involving more than 1 tendon and at least 4 cm long in the sagittal plane, and group IV being massive tears with osteoarthritis of the humeral head. Cofield and colleagues[2] defined a massive rotator cuff tear as a tear of 5 cm or more. Burkhart[3] used a similar definition of a massive tear as one that is at least 5 cm long with no superior coverage, referred to by Rockwood[4] as a "bald head." Gerber and colleagues[5] commented that there was no universal agreement on the definition of a massive tear, and believed that it was more appropriate to describe the tear in terms of the amount of tendon that has been detached from the tuberosities rather than as a discrete number such as 5 cm, because of variations in patient size and techniques of measurement. He defined a rotator cuff tear as massive if it involved the detachment of at least 2 entire tendons, noting that most massive tears involve the supraspinatus and infraspinatus, but that anterosuperior tears involving the supraspinatus and subscapularis also occur with moderate frequency. Warner and colleagues[6] supported use of Gerber and colleagues' definition as a more functional definition than one based on a simple measurement of the length of the tear, because an exact measurement of the length of the tear can be made only after the edges of degenerative tendon tissue have been debrided. These investigators also point out that a massive tear is not necessarily irreparable, and an irreparable tear is not always massive. In a separate article, Warner and Parsons[7] described an irreparable tear as one characterized by the inability to achieve a direct repair of native tendon to the proximal humerus despite mobilization of the remaining tissue with conventional techniques of soft tissue release. These tears are often chronic in nature and result in attritional changes in both the tendon substance and muscle fibers. Acute massive tears may be larger than 5 cm but may have tendon that is good quality and easily repaired to its anatomic insertion. Conversely, a small chronic tear may have thin, inelastic, friable tissue that is impossible to mobilize and repair. According to Warner,[6] an acromiohumeral distance less than 5 mm (**Fig. 1**A) usually means that the tear involves at least 2 tendons of the rotator

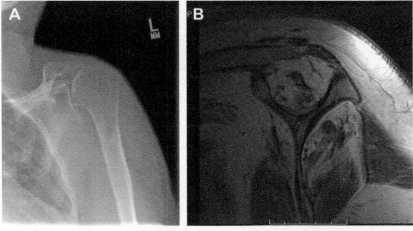

Fig. 1. (*A*) True anteroposterior radiograph showing superior migration of the humeral head and decreased acromiohumeral distance. (*B*) Sagittal T1 image of the same patient with severe Goutallier grade IV fatty degeneration of the subscapularis, supraspinatus, and infraspinatus.

cuff, and this in combination with magnetic resonance imaging (MRI) showing severe muscle atrophy with advanced fatty degeneration of the muscles (see **Fig. 1**B) indicates an irreparable tear. He notes that fewer than 5% of rotator cuff tears remain irreparable, attributed to poor tissue quality as much as tear size.

Limited nonarthroplasty surgical options exist for the treatment of irreparable rotator cuff tears. Debridement of the tear, open or arthroscopic, and acromioplasty may be appropriate under certain circumstances, such as for the low-demand patient.[8-11] Burkhart and colleagues[12] have shown that partial repair of massive irreparable rotator cuff tears can result in dramatic improvement in function when the normal mechanics of the shoulder are restored, rather than striving to achieve full coverage of the defect. The long head of biceps tendon has been implicated as a source of pain in irreparable rotator cuff tears, and therefore there can be a role for biceps tenotomy in treatment of this disorder.[13] Rotator cuff augmentation with allografts or extracellular matrix scaffolds, such as acellular human dermis and small intestinal submucosa, has shown mixed results, and level 1 evidence is lacking.[14-16]

Suprascapular neuropathy (SSN) has been shown to be a potential neurogenic cause of pain with massive rotator cuff tear. Boykin and colleagues[17] have shown that SSN, as proved on electrodiagnostic studies, is more frequent in patients with massive rotator cuff tears, and Lafosse and colleagues[18] have reported positive results of arthroscopic decompression of the nerve in this population. Partial repair of a massive rotator cuff tear may change the tension on the nerve, and may be another mechanism of pain relief in SSN.[19,20]

Tendon transfers may be an option in appropriate patients. Patients without glenohumeral arthritis but with marked weakness and pain in the setting of a massive, irreparable rotator cuff tear can benefit from a tendon transfer. Latissimus dorsi transfer to reconstruct a massive posterosuperior rotator cuff tear was originally developed by Gerber.[21] Patients with functional impairment who may also have loss of external rotation strength can be considered for this procedure if they do not have pseudoparalysis. Pectoralis major transfer has been used in some cases to reconstruct an irreparable subscapularis tear.[22]

In this review, we provide evidence-based guidelines for nonarthroplasty options in the treatment of massive, irreparable rotator cuff tears. Most of the available evidence is level IV evidence, because prospective controlled studies are rare and generally not feasible, or in many cases unethical, for surgical studies. The American Academy of Orthopaedic Surgeons (AAOS) clinical practice guideline on optimizing the management of rotator cuff problems was of limited usefulness because of the lack of strong recommendations; the 1 guideline dealing specifically with irreparable rotator cuff tears, which stated that it is an option to perform partial rotator cuff repair, debridement, or muscle transfers for patients with irreparable rotator cuff tears when surgery is indicated, had a strength of recommendation that was graded as weak.[23] It is important to consider each patient as an individual, both in terms of their expectations and functional demands, as well as their ability to undergo intensive rehabilitation protocols, before deciding which treatment course to embark upon. This is a concept referred to by Patte[1]: that one must consider the patient's somatotype, age, social and professional activities, and degree of expected cooperation in the postoperative period when thinking about the prognosis of an individual shoulder with a rotator cuff tear.

DEBRIDEMENT AND SUBACROMIAL DECOMPRESSION

The relief of pain as the primary goal in surgery for the massive rotator cuff tear led to considerable interest in debridement of massive, irreparable rotator cuff tears combined with some type of acromioplasty or subacromial decompression, without necessarily attempting to repair the rotator cuff tear. This approach may not yield functional benefit in terms of strength and range of motion, but can provide significant benefit in terms of pain relief, particularly in the lower-demand patient. In addition, there may be secondary functional gains related to decreased pain. However, function generally is not restored, and the effectiveness of this treatment may be limited.[24]

Hawkins and colleagues[9] described a series of 100 consecutive patients with full-thickness rotator cuff tears who underwent anteroinferior partial acromioplasty as described by Neer.[25] Twenty-seven of these patients had massive tears, defined as greater than 5 cm. Only 6 patients had tears that were deemed irreparable. The investigators describe performing extensive debridement in these 6 patients, with resection of bursal tissue and anterior acromioplasty. Although the irreparable tears were not analyzed separately, all patients had relief of pain postoperatively. The tear size was correlated to outcome, in that the smaller the tear, the more likely the recovery of strength and decrease in pain.

The status of the deltoid in determining the outcome after debridement of a massive rotator cuff tear was highlighted by Rockwood and colleagues[11] All of the patients in this series had irreparable rotator cuff tears treated with open modified Neer acromioplasty, subacromial decompression, including resection of the coracoacromial ligament (CAL), and debridement of massive tears involving supraspinatus and infraspinatus. At 6.5-year follow-up, 83% of the 50 patients had satisfactory results. The investigators noted that favorable results were obtained if the anterior deltoid was preserved and if there had been no previous acromioplasty or attempt at rotator cuff repair. They suggested that the pain relief seen postoperatively was a result of adequate subacromial decompression and the preserved functional range of motion was caused by strength in the anterior deltoid and in the remaining subscapularis and teres minor muscles, which was regained through a detailed rehabilitation program. These results suggest that, with proper rehabilitation, adequate decompression of the subacromial space, anterior acromioplasty, and debridement of massive tears of the rotator cuff can lead to the relief of pain and the restoration of function.

In Rockwood and colleagues' series, the superior portion of the subscapularis or teres minor was rarely involved in the tear. When the subscapularis and teres minor are intact, normal function in the face of unrepaired, massive tears of the supraspinatus and infraspinatus can still occur. This situation is because of the preservation of the force couples in the transverse and coronal planes, as explained by Burkhart.[3]

With the advancement of arthroscopy, open debridement and acromioplasty have largely been replaced by arthroscopic methods. Gartsman[8] described 154 shoulders treated with arthroscopic subacromial decompression and no attempt to repair the rotator cuff tear. Twenty-five of these patients had full-thickness tears; however, only 3 of these tears were classified as massive. An important correlation was seen between the final result and the size of the tear. Thirteen of the 16 patients with a tear measuring less than 3 cm had a satisfactory result, but only 1 of the 9 patients with a tear greater than 3 cm had a satisfactory result, and 8 of these 9 patients went on to further operative treatment. Gartsman concluded that results were unsatisfactory in patients with a massive rotator cuff tear.

The correlation between tear size and results after subacromial decompression was again shown by Levy and colleagues.[10] Of 25 patients treated with arthroscopic subacromial decompression for full-thickness rotator cuff tears, all had significantly decreased pain postoperatively but small tears fared better than large tears. In a follow-up study of the same patients, Zvijac and colleagues[26] emphasized that results of subacromial decompression and debridement of full-thickness rotator cuff tears deteriorated over time. Large and massive tears fared worse over time than small and moderate tears. The conclusions drawn were that for repairable tears, subacromial decompression and debridement could not be recommended over repair of the rotator cuff, but for select patients with irreparable tears, it may have a role. Melillo and Savoie[24] agreed with this conclusion in their comparative study of open repair versus debridement of massive rotator cuff tears, stating that results of debridement deteriorate significantly with time and are not acceptable.

This theory was echoed by Ellman and colleagues,[27] who stated that arthroscopic subacromial decompression and debridement of full-thickness rotator cuff tears has a valuable, but limited, role in carefully selected patients. They noted that patients with massive, irreparable tears did not regain strength or range of motion, but did have significant pain relief.

Looking specifically at patients with massive, irreparable rotator cuff tears, Gartsman[28] reported on a series of 33 patients. All patients had at least a 5-cm tear involving 2 or more tendons that could not be repaired without excessive tension. Open debridement and subacromial decompression led to a significant decrease in pain and an increase in range of motion and ability to perform activities of daily living. Gartsman noted that strength in elevation was decreased postoperatively. The results were inferior to rotator cuff repair. However, comparison with patients with tears that were possible to repair may not be reasonable, because patients with massive, irreparable tears are generally older, may have a biceps tear or superior migration of the humeral head, and often have poorer-quality muscle and tendon tissue.

To better compare open repair and arthroscopic debridement of full-thickness rotator cuff tears, Montgomery and colleagues[29] randomized 88 shoulders to receive one of these treatments. Although no distinction was made between reparable and irreparable tears, 50% of the debridement group and 28% of the repair group had massive rotator cuff tears (>5 cm). Within each group, results were better in younger patients with smaller tears, but this did not reach statistical significance. Five of 19 patients in the debridement group went on to develop cuff tear arthropathy and were treated with hemiarthroplasty. The investigators concluded that arthroscopic debridement and subacromial decompression was inferior to rotator cuff repair. Size of tear, patient age, or activity level did not correlate with the results achieved by arthroscopic debridement, and it was not possible to identify any consistent parameters that would define a group of patients who would do well with arthroscopic debridement alone.

In his series of 10 shoulders with massive rotator cuff tears treated with arthroscopic acromioplasty and rotator cuff debridement, Burkhart reported that normal shoulder function was possible with a massive, unrepaired rotator cuff tear.[3] This was a subset of patients whose only activity-limiting factor was pain. Open rotator cuff repair was avoided because it was believed that this would result in an unacceptable loss of range of motion. All patients had a massive tear, defined as greater than 5 cm with no superior coverage, and none had preoperative superior migration of the humeral head. All 10 achieved pain relief without loss of motion or strength, at a mean follow-up of 18 months. Burkhart emphasizes 2 important force couples as the key factor in predicting success of debridement and subacromial decompression. The first force couple is that in the coronal plane between the deltoid and the inferior rotator cuff. The second force couple is in the transverse plane between the anterior cuff (subscapularis) and the posterior cuff (infraspinatus and teres minor). Normal function in the face of an unrepaired rotator cuff tear can still be achieved, but only if these force couples remain intact. (**Fig. 2**). This balance depends on the integrity of the anterior cuff, the posterior cuff, and the deltoid. Most massive rotator cuff tears extend to

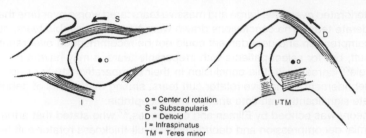

o = Center of rotation
S = Subscapularis
D = Deltoid
I = Infraspinatus
TM = Teres minor

Fig. 2. Uncoupling of either essential force couple results in loss of ability to maintain a fulcrum for motion at the glenohumeral joint. (*Reprinted from* Burkhart SS. Arthroscopic treatment of massive rotator cuff tears. Clin Orthop Rel Res 1991;267:52; with permission.)

involve the posterior cuff, and involvement of subscapularis is less common, therefore the crucial point in determining whether to repair the rotator cuff is the status of the posterior rotator cuff. In a massive tear, the posterior cuff may be torn so badly that it is unable to balance the moment created anteriorly by subscapularis, which then leads to inability to maintain the equilibrium of the glenohumeral fulcrum in the transverse plane. This situation can cause such a decrease in the moment developed by the inferior cuff that it can no longer maintain equilibrium in the coronal plane, giving a net effect of anterior-superior translation of the humeral head with attempted elevation. An intact posterior cuff is the key to successful treatment by arthroscopic acromioplasty and debridement. Burkhart found that strength of resisted external rotation was a reliable preoperative indicator of intact posterior cuff. Furthermore, Burkhart stated that the dynamic transverse and coronal plane force couples, as outlined earlier, are more important than any passive constraint or humeral head depressing action provided by the long head of the biceps.

Wiley[30] described superior humeral head migration as a complication of rotator cuff debridement and bursal decompression in a case series of 4 patients. Two of these patients had undergone hemiarthroplasty for fracture, and in these patients it was the prosthesis that migrated superiorly. In all 4 patients, attempts had been made to repair the massive rotator cuff tear. In every case, the CAL had been divided. In 2 patients, bone graft was used to reestablish the subacromial arch from the coracoid process to the undersurface of the acromion, with good pain relief and correction of deformity. Wiley concluded that debridement alone may lead to upward dislocation of the humeral head and an increase in disability.

The issue of superior humeral head migration and the importance of the coracoacromial arch was further explored by subsequent investigators. Fagelman and colleagues[31] performed a cadaveric study on 7 shoulders. A significant decrease in anterosuperior migration was found after CAL reconstruction compared with both anterior acromioplasty and modified Neer acromioplasty. The investigators deduced that in patients with massive rotator cuff tears, reconstruction of the CAL may provide the necessary stabilizing force to prevent excessive anterosuperior translation and possible humeral head escape from the coracoacromial arch. They suggest that only minimal bone should be resected when performing acromioplasty, and the CAL should be preserved when possible. They also recommend that when CAL preservation is not possible, anatomic reconstruction of the medial band of the CAL is warranted in patients with coracoacromial arch deficiency. Flatow and colleagues[32] examined CAL reconstruction in vivo in a series of 16 patients undergoing repair of a massive rotator cuff tear. The CAL was repaired with bone sutures to the acromion.

Of 10 patients available for follow-up, 8 had satisfactory results and were able to perform overhead activities. Two had unsatisfactory results. There were no cases of anterosuperior humeral head subluxation. Although these were not irreparable rotator cuff tears, this series shows that acromioplasty with CAL preservation or repair maintains some of the passive stabilizing effect of the coracoacromial arch.

In 2002, Fenlin and colleagues[33] introduced a new procedure for treatment of massive, irreparable rotator cuff tears that facilitated CAL preservation. This procedure was described as a tuberoplasty, which involves removal of exostoses on the humerus followed by reshaping of the greater tuberosity to create a smooth, congruent acromiohumeral articulation. The CAL is preserved and an acromioplasty is not performed. The investigators reported on 20 patients with a minimum of 27 months follow-up, all of whom had disabling pain preoperatively. All patients had a tear of at least 5 cm involving both supraspinatus and infraspinatus (2 also had partial subscapularis tears). In all cases, rotator cuff repair was abandoned because of excessive retraction or poor tissue quality after mobilization, or both. In the tuberoplasty procedure, the acromion and CAL are left intact until a decision is made about the reparability of the cuff. The investigators emphasize that it is vital to make this determination before violating the coracoacromial arch. There were 12 excellent results, 6 good, and 1 fair. Sixty-eight percent of patients were totally pain free and no patient had night pain postoperatively. All patients had residual external rotation weakness. These results, although clearly showing improvements in pain and function, are still inferior to results achieved with acromioplasty and repair of the rotator cuff. The investigators conclude that despite the role of the acromion and CAL in the pathogenesis of impingement syndrome, its importance in a select group of patients with massive, irreparable rotator cuff tears cannot be overemphasized.

Debridement of massive rotator cuff tears and subacromial decompression, although overall inferior to repair of the rotator cuff when possible, may still have a role in elderly, low-demand patients for whom pain relief is the priority and functional goals are limited. Results have been shown to deteriorate over time. Satisfactory results are most likely to be achieved in patients in whom the integrity of the deltoid is preserved and who have good external rotation strength preoperatively, indicating an intact posterior rotator cuff.

PARTIAL REPAIR, MARGIN CONVERGENCE

Burkhart[34] coined the term margin convergence to describe side-to-side closure of massive, U-shaped rotator cuff tears. He recognized that most massive rotator cuff tears are not retracted but are L-shaped tears with a vertical split from medial to lateral, which assume a U shape because of the elasticity of the muscle-tendon unit. Burkhart cited McLaughlin as advocating a repair that used a combination of side-to-side tendon-to-tendon sutures and end-on tendon-to-bone sutures in the 1940s. Furthermore, Burkhart stated that mobilization of these tears leads to failure of repair because of tension overload at the apex of the tear, whereas side-to-side closure gives a mechanical advantage because of a biomechanical principle called margin convergence. In the technique of margin convergence, the free margin of the tear converges toward the greater tuberosity as side-to-side repair progresses (**Figs. 3** and **4**). As the margin converges, the strain at the free edge of the cuff is reduced significantly, leaving an almost tension-free converged cuff margin overlying the humeral bone bed for repair. Side-to-side closure of two-thirds of a U-shaped tear reduces the strain at the cuff margin to one-sixth of the strain that existed at the pre-converged cuff margin. This strategy gives a lower probability of failure of fixation to

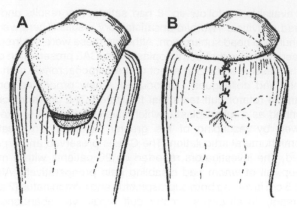

Fig. 3. (*A*) U-shaped rotator cuff tear. (*B*) Partial side-to-side repair causes a margin convergence of the tear toward the greater tuberosity, which increases the cross-sectional area and decreases the length of the tear, thereby decreasing strain. (*Reprinted from* Burkhart SS. Arthroscopic treatment of massive rotator cuff tears. Clin Orthop Rel Res 2001;390:109; with permission.)

bone, either by anchors or transosseous tunnels. The principles of margin convergence and force couples must be followed when attempting repair of a massive rotator cuff tear. Partial repair, in which there is a defect remaining in the superior portion of the cuff after margin convergence, can still be effective, if at least half of the infraspinatus can be repaired to bone. Burkhart recommends partial repair

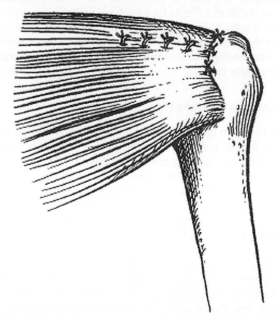

Fig. 4. After placing side-to-side sutures, the free margin of the cuff is repaired to bone with suture anchors. (*Reprinted from* Burkhart SS. Arthroscopic treatment of massive rotator cuff tears. Clin Orthop Rel Res 2001;390:114; with permission.)

whenever complete closure of the defect is not possible, and advises against local transfers of rotator cuff tendons. In truly nonmobile tears, an interval slide as described by Tauro[35] sometimes allows an additional 1 to 2 cm of lateral excursion of the supraspinatus tendon and therefore permits a greater degree of partial repair. The results of this technique are variable.

Partial repair has been studied in a rat model by Hsu and colleagues[36] comparing no repair, infraspinatus repair, or 2-tendon repair 4 weeks after detachment of infraspinatus and supraspinatus in 48 rats. Quantitative ambulatory measures performed in each group (medial/lateral forces, braking, propulsion, step width) were significantly different between the no repair group and the infraspinatus repair group, and were similar between the infraspinatus and the 2-tendon repair groups. The investigators concluded that repairing the infraspinatus back to its insertion site without repair of the supraspinatus can improve shoulder function to a similar extent as repairing both infraspinatus and supraspinatus.

Mazzocca and colleagues[37] examined in a cadaveric study whether there was biomechanical rationale for performing margin convergence in large, retracted rotator cuff tears. Twenty cadaveric shoulders in which the supraspinatus muscle-tendon unit was removed to create a large retracted rotator cuff tear were tested. Margin convergence was performed in an open fashion by placing simple sutures 5 mm apart beginning at the glenoid rim medially and proceeding laterally. Gap area was measured after each suture was placed. There was a statistically significant gap closure with each suture: 50% with the first suture, 60% with the second suture, 67% with the third suture, and 75% with the fourth suture ($P<.05$). Infraspinatus and supraspinatus strain were measured for each specimen in the intact state, after supraspinatus removal, after each convergence suture was placed, and in different positions of rotation and abduction. When comparing infraspinatus strain and subscapularis strain before and after margin convergence was performed, the investigators found that strain was significantly reduced at all degrees of rotation in 0° of abduction after margin convergence sutures were placed ($P<.05$). Testing was also conducted to calculate glenohumeral joint translation and to measure tension in the rotator cuff itself during knot tying and gap closure. The investigators found that there was minimal tension and stress in the rotator cuff during knot tying. Infraspinatus and subscapularis strain increased slightly as the tendons were pulled together during knot tying. The first margin convergence suture caused the greatest increase in intrinsic rotator cuff tension, with each subsequent suture having a similar but less dramatic effect. Overall, mean anterior translation of the humeral head was minimal. The results obtained support the hypothesis that margin convergence decreases the size of the tear gap and reduces strain with minimal effect on glenohumeral translation and intrinsic tendon strain during knot tying.

BICEPS TENOTOMY AND TENODESIS

Patte[1] alluded to the relevance of the long head of the biceps in his proposed system of classification of rotator cuff tears. Walch[13] observed in the late 1980s that many patients with chronic rotator cuff tears experience pain relief after rupturing the long head of the biceps, once the acute episode subsides. He therefore hypothesized that selected patients with chronic rotator cuff tears may benefit from tenotomy of the long head of biceps. He subsequently reported long-term follow-up (2–14 years) on 307 patients with full-thickness rotator cuff tears treated with tenotomy of the long head of the biceps. All patients had symmetric passive range of motion with the contralateral shoulder. Patients were selected for biceps tenotomy if the rotator cuff tear was irreparable, or if the patient was older and unwilling to undergo the rehabilitation required after rotator cuff repair. There was a significant improvement in mean Constant score from 48.4 to 67.6 after biceps tenotomy, and 87% of patients were satisfied or very satisfied with their result. The acromiohumeral distance decreased by 1.3 mm during the follow-up period, and was associated with a longer duration of follow-up. Preoperatively 38% of patients had glenohumeral arthritis, at latest follow-up 67% had arthritis. Only patients with an acromiohumeral interval of greater than 6 mm gained a statistically significant benefit from concomitant acromioplasty. Teres minor atrophy in patients with fatty infiltration of infraspinatus was found to negatively influence many clinical and radiographic outcome parameters. In multivariate regression analysis, the 3 factors found to most influence postoperative adjusted Constant scores were: preoperative adjusted Constant score, fatty infiltration of the subscapularis muscle, and fatty infiltration of the infraspinatus muscle. One percent of patients underwent subsequent rotator cuff repair, and 2% of patients underwent later surgery for cuff tear arthropathy. No cosmetic deformity as a result of biceps tenotomy was identifiable in approximately half of patients. No patient rated their result as fair or poor because of cosmesis. The investigators conclude that in selected patients, biceps tenotomy for rotator cuff tears leads to good objective outcomes and high patient satisfaction. They note that it does not alter the progressive degenerative radiographic changes in the glenohumeral joint that are seen with chronic rotator cuff tears.

Boileau and colleagues[38] again showed that biceps tenotomy can lead to symptomatic improvement in massive rotator cuff tears, and also showed that biceps tenodesis has the same benefits. In this study, 39 irreparable rotator cuff tears were treated with arthroscopic tenotomy of the long head of biceps and 33 irreparable tears were treated with arthroscopic biceps tenodesis. Tenodesis was preferentially performed in more active patients and in those less than the age of 65 years. At a mean follow-up of 35 months, 78% of patients were satisfied with the result. The mean Constant score improved from 46.3 to 66.5. There were 3 patients with pseudoparalysis, and these patients did not benefit from the procedure. None of them regained active forward elevation above horizontal. In contrast, the 15 patients with painful loss of active elevation recovered active elevation. The investigators emphasize the importance, therefore, of differentiating between pseudoparalysis and painful loss of active elevation. They furthermore state that pseudoparalysis and severe cuff tear arthropathy are contraindications to biceps tenotomy or tenodesis as a treatment of massive rotator cuff tear. Two patients in this series went on to have reverse total shoulder arthroplasty. Sixty-two percent of patients with a biceps tenotomy developed a cosmetic deformity but only 16 patients were aware of the deformity and none was bothered by it. Similar to Walch, Boileau found that absence or atrophy of the teres minor on preoperative imaging was associated with severe fatty infiltration of the infraspinatus and with significant decreases in both postoperative external rotation and the postoperative Constant score. Given the influence of the status of the teres minor on final outcomes, Boileau's group now performs an additional latissimus dorsi and teres major transfer when a patient has a severe external rotation deficit with a teres minor that is torn or has fatty infiltration, and the goal is more than simple palliation or pain relief.

SSN IN ASSOCIATION WITH MASSIVE ROTATOR CUFF TEARS

There has been increasing interest in recent years in the role of the suprascapular nerve in shoulder pain, particularly when associated with massive rotator cuff tears.

Warner and colleagues[39] published a detailed account in 1992 of the anatomy and relationships of the suprascapular nerve. This was a cadaver study to delineate the anatomic relationships of the suprascapular nerve and to define the dangers to this structure with mobilization of a massive rotator cuff tear. One hypothesis was that unexplained clinical failures of lateral advancement techniques used in treatment of massive rotator cuff tears may have been caused by extensive mobilization causing damage to the neurovascular pedicle to the supraspinatus and infraspinatus. In this study, 31 cadaver shoulders were dissected. In all shoulders, the suprascapular nerve was found to be closely applied to the bony floor of the supraspinatus fossa and was tethered at the suprascapular notch deep to the transverse scapular ligament. Tension on the motor branches was assessed visually and by palpation after disinsertion and advancement of the supraspinatus and infraspinatus. When any motor branch became so taut that it could not be moved from side to side, or became avulsed from the muscle, this was considered the limit to lateral transposition of the muscle. In 5 shoulders, the amount of mobilization of the cuff that is safely possible through an anterosuperior approach and detachment of the deltoid was assessed. This amount was found to be 1 cm. In 8 shoulders, a modified advancement technique in which the muscle was advanced laterally within a subperiosteally elevated fascial sleeve was evaluated. Using this technique, neither the supraspinatus nor infraspinatus could be advanced laterally by more than 3 cm. In all shoulders, the limiting factor for lateral advancement of supraspinatus and infraspinatus was tension on the motor branches of the suprascapular nerve. In most shoulders, lateral advancement of the muscle caused the first motor branch of the suprascapular nerve to become kinked under the ligament in the notch. In these shoulders, release of the ligament resulted in an additional 5 mm of lateral advancement of the tendon before the nerve came under tension. The investigators noted that when a tendon has retracted in a chronic rotator cuff tear, the neurovascular bundle may be tethered by scar tissue and may be at even greater risk than suggested by this study (**Fig. 5**). It was shown that the maximum lateral advancement of the cuff that is permitted by the neurovascular structures is 3 cm, which is less than what is usually required for repair of massive tears of

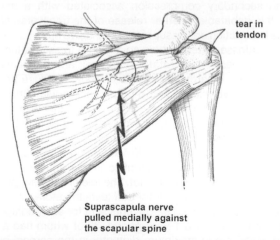

tear in
tendon

Suprascapula nerve
pulled medially against
the scapular spine

Fig. 5. Tethering of the suprascapular nerve with progressive medial retraction of large rotator cuff tendon tears. (*Reprinted from* Costouros JG, Porramatikul M, Lie DT, et al. Reversal of suprascapular neuropathy following arthroscopic repair of massive supraspinatus and infraspinatus rotator cuff tears. Arthroscopy 2007;23(11):1153; with permission.)

the rotator cuff. This situation may explain failure of supraspinatus or infraspinatus to regain strength after repair of massive rotator cuff tear.

Vad and colleagues[40] examined the prevalence of peripheral nerve injury associated with rotator cuff tears with atrophy and found that 7 of 25 patients with full-thickness rotator cuff tears had abnormal electromyographic (EMG) studies. Of these 7 patients, 2 had SSN. Mallon and colleagues[20] reported on a prospective, consecutive series of 8 patients with massive (>5 cm) rotator cuff tears with fatty infiltration and retraction of supraspinatus on MRI. All 8 patients had SSN on EMG. Four patients underwent debridement and partial repair, 2 of whom underwent follow-up EMG, which showed in both cases that the suprascapular nerve had significant renervation potentials, with almost complete recovery of the nerve in 1 case.

Costouros and colleagues[19] showed reversal of SSN in patients with massive rotator cuff tears after partial or complete repair. Twenty-six of 216 patients with rotator cuff tears treated operatively were identified to have massive tears associated with retraction and moderate to severe fatty infiltration of the supraspinatus and infraspinatus muscles. Fourteen of these patients were found to have a peripheral nerve injury on EMG, of whom 7 had an isolated suprascapular nerve injury. All 7 underwent arthroscopic treatment of their rotator cuff tear. One tear was not technically reparable at time of surgery. In the 6 patients who underwent either partial or complete arthroscopic repair, follow-up EMG/nerve conduction velocities after 6 months showed partial or full recovery of the suprascapular nerve palsy, which correlated with complete pain relief and marked improvement in function. Although numbers were small, this study suggests that repair or partial repair of the massive rotator cuff tear, by relieving the traction on the suprascapular nerve, may alleviate the associated SSN without performing direct decompression of the nerve at the time of surgery.

In 2007, Lafosse and colleagues[18] described a novel, all-arthroscopic technique for decompressing the suprascapular nerve, initially in patients without rotator cuff tears. There is believed to be less postoperative scar formation and fibrosis after an arthroscopic procedure compared with open decompression and, subsequently, less risk of recurrent nerve compression. In a subsequent review article, Lafosse and colleagues[41] discussed the distinction between primary suprascapular nerve compression and secondary compression associated with a massive, retracted rotator cuff tear. It is debatable whether release of the transverse scapular ligament is necessary once the traction on the suprascapular nerve has been relieved by repairing the rotator cuff. Lafosse states that his approach is to assess the nerve, the notch and the transverse ligament during rotator cuff repair and to release a thickened or ossified ligament (**Fig. 6**), regardless of EMG findings, because he believes arthroscopic suprascapular nerve release is a safe procedure with little risk of additional complications. He cites his unpublished series of 75 patients with massive rotator cuff tear who had rotator cuff repair, in whom associated SSN in 29 (39%) was identified by positive EMG preoperatively. All 29 patients underwent an EMG at 6 months postoperatively, of whom 13 had normal EMG, 12 had improvement, and 4 had no change. No statistical difference was identified in this small group between those who had nerve release and those who did not. The role of suprascapular nerve decompression in management of massive rotator cuff tears therefore remains controversial.

Boykin and colleagues[17] reviewed 92 patients sent for electrodiagnostic evaluation of the suprascapular nerve over a 1-year period, 38 of whom had a massive rotator cuff tear (defined as ≥5 cm in maximum diameter in the coronal or sagittal plane). Of the patients with an electrodiagnosis of SSN, 23 patients had a massive rotator cuff tear, 2 had a full-thickness tear not considered massive, and 15 did not have rotator cuff disease. The likelihood of SSN was greater among patients with a massive

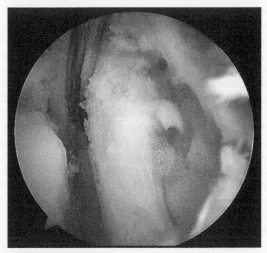

Fig. 6. Arthroscopic image of an ossified transverse ligament of the left shoulder.

rotator cuff tear (60.5% [23/38]) than patients without a massive cuff tear (31.5% [17/54], P<.05). The investigators believed that the mechanism of injury to the SSN in this situation was traction from retraction of the rotator cuff musculature. The prevalence of SSN among patients with a massive cuff tear was lower in those patients who had previous attempted rotator cuff repair compared with those without previous repair, but this did not reach statistical significance. The investigators also comment that although the suprascapular nerve was previously considered a solely motor nerve, there is increasing evidence that it has a sensory component that can be a major contributor to shoulder pain. This concept is supported by the fact that suprascapular nerve blocks have been shown to significantly decrease pain after shoulder surgery. The investigators conclude that whether rotator cuff repair in the presence of SSN is adequate without additional decompression of the nerve will be answered only in comparative trials.

TENDON TRANSFERS

Irreparable tears can be defined as those in which direct tendon-to-bone repair and healing are not possible. Tendon transfers have gained acceptance as a treatment option for this situation. Local tendon transposition, distant tendon transfer, and deltoid flap transposition have all been proposed as methods of reconstructing the rotator cuff. Use of a portion of subscapularis and teres major to cover superior cuff defects has been used with limited success, and results were not reproducible.[42] Distant tendon transfer in the form of latissimus dorsi transfer for massive posterosuperior tears and pectoralis major transfers for the less common anterosuperior tears have had more reproducible and long-term success.

Latissimus Dorsi Transfer

Latissimus dorsi transfer was proposed by Gerber and colleagues in 1988[43] to reconstruct tears involving complete loss of supraspinatus and infraspinatus. They described transfer of the latissimus dorsi tendon from its insertion on the humeral shaft to the superolateral humeral head. Converting teres major and latissimus dorsi into external rotators had been previously shown by l'Episcopo[44] to be effective in children with brachial plexus birth palsies. Gerber viewed massive rotator cuff tears as an analogous adult problem. The latissimus dorsi provides a large, vascularized tendon to close the rotator cuff defect. The transfer of latissimus dorsi to the superolateral humeral head converts latissimus dorsi to a humeral head depressor by virtue of its almost vertical orientation, and into an external rotator by virtue of its insertion relative to the humeral head. It was noted from the outset that this procedure was not designed for shoulders with poor deltoid function. Gerber and colleagues first dissected 12 cadaver shoulders to define the relevant anatomy, and to confirm that the tendon was sufficient to cover at least part of the cuff defect, the length of tendon enough to allow transfer to superolateral humeral head and to allow good range of motion of the shoulder after transfer, and that the neurovascular pedicle was constant and long enough to allow the transfer without tension on the neurovascular structures. Transfer of the latissimus dorsi to the humeral head was easily possible in all 12 cadaveric shoulders. The investigators then applied the technique to 14 patients with massive rotator cuff tears, 9 of whom had a severe functional handicap. The rotator cuff could be closed with the aid of latissimus dorsi in 10 of the 14 cases. Postoperative EMGs in the first 11 patients confirmed normal suprascapular and thoracodorsal nerve function, as well as showing that one of the patients had innervated latissimus dorsi during shoulder flexion and 3 of the patients on external rotation. EMG studies suggested that the latissimus dorsi acted mainly by tenodesis to produce external rotation. Gerber's initial series showed promising results at 1-year follow-up, with gains in forward flexion, abduction, control of external rotation in abduction, and a decrease in fatigability of the shoulder for patients using their arm between waist and shoulder level. Gerber did not transfer teres major with latissimus dorsi because the teres major is often too bulky to pass under the deltoid, and because the amplitude and the length of the teres major tendon was considered insufficient.

In a later study of 69 shoulders with massive, irreparable rotator cuff tears, Gerber showed that long-term results of latissimus dorsi transfer were positive.[45] At mean follow-up of 53 months, average subjective shoulder value had increased from 28% preoperatively to 66% postoperatively. The mean age and gender-matched Constant and Murley score improved from 55% to 73% (P<.0001). The pain score improved from 6 to 12 points (of a possible 15 points) (P<.0001). Flexion increased from 104° to 123°, abduction increased from 101° to 119°, and external rotation increased from 22° to 29° (P<.05). Strength increased from 0.9 to 1.8 kg (P<.0001). Thirteen patients had deficient subscapularis preoperatively, as evidenced by a positive liftoff test. These patients did not achieve the improvements in function and pain seen by those with an intact subscapularis. Gerber concluded that latissimus dorsi transfer durably and substantially improves chronically painful, dysfunctional shoulders with irreparable rotator cuff tears, especially if the subscapularis is intact, but that if subscapularis function is deficient, the procedure is of questionable benefit and probably should not be used.

In an anatomic study of 18 cadavers, Morelli and colleagues[46] defined the critical anatomy for latissimus dorsi tendon harvest. They emphasized the landmark of a deep fibrous band at the confluence of teres major and latissimus dorsi (**Fig. 7**), and reported that the radial nerve crosses from ventral to dorsal directly beneath the latissimus dorsi, 22.1 mm (standard deviation 3.6 mm) deep to this band, and 36.5 mm (standard deviation 12.7) from the tendon insertion on the humerus, whereas the axillary nerve exits the quadrangular space 27 mm (8.9) from the humeral insertion of latissimus dorsi and teres major (**Table 1**).

The investigators found that the distance from the latissimus dorsi insertion on the humerus to its neurovascular pedicle was 110.3 mm (standard deviation 13.7). They

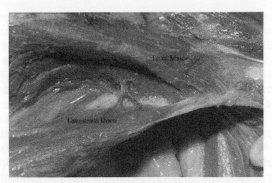

Fig. 7. The confluence of teres major and latissimus dorsi where the deep fibrous band forms (relevant anatomy to latissimus dorsi transfer). (*Reprinted from* Morelli M, Nagamori J, Gilbart M, et al. Latissimus dorsi transfer for massive irreparable cuff tears: an anatomic study. J Shoulder Elbow Surg 2008;17:141; with permission.)

concluded that harvest of the latissimus dorsi tendon can be safely accomplished by identifying the deep fibrous band and releasing the tendon within 2 cm of its humeral attachment.

Ianotti and colleagues[47] found that preoperative shoulder function and general strength influence the outcome after latissimus dorsi transfer. In their study of 14 patients undergoing latissimus dorsi transfer for massive rotator cuff tear, women with poor shoulder function had a greater probability of a poor clinical result. The investigators reported that the most significant predictors of outcome were preoperative active range of motion, and strength in forward flexion and external rotation. The transfer does not overcome pseudoparalysis.

Latissimus dorsi transfer as a salvage procedure after failed rotator cuff repair has been shown to be effective. Miniaci and MacLeod[48] studied 17 such patients, at

Table 1
Anatomic landmarks of significance for latissimus dorsi transfer

Landmark	Distance (mm) (Mean ± SD)	Range (mm)
Inferior angle of scapula to superior border of LD	20.6 ± 9.5	5–44
Inferior angle of scapula to lateral border of LD	81.4 ± 9.5	48–120
Inferior angle of scapula to DFB	113.9 ± 16.6	91–153
DFB to LD tendon insertion into humerus	36.5 ± 12.7	10–56
Width of LD tendon at insertion into humerus	33.1 ± 7.5	22–48
Length of LD tendon	51.8 ± 11.1	27–74
Narrowest width of LD tendon	24.5 ± 5.2	18–35
Length of TM tendon	9.0 ± 7.6	0–20
Width of TM tendon	34.1 ± 7.7	19–48

No statistical difference was noted between extremities with paired *t* testing for each of the items listed.

Abbreviations: DFB, deep fibrous band; LD, latissimus dorsi; SD, standard deviation; TM, teres major.

Reprinted from Morelli M, Nagamori J, Gilbart M, et al. Latissimus dorsi transfer for massive irreparable cuff tears: an anatomic study. J Shoulder Elbow Surg 2008;17:140.

a mean follow-up of 51 months. Six of their patients had undergone more than 1 previous attempted rotator cuff repair. After latissimus dorsi transfer, 14 of the 17 patients had significant pain relief and improvement in function for all activities except lifting heavier than 6.8 kg (15 pounds). Both active and the passive range of motion improved in forward elevation and in internal and external rotation ($P<.0001$). Seven of 8 patients with a detached or nonfunctioning anterior deltoid had substantial improvement. The investigators could not detect any significant differences, either preoperatively or postoperatively, between patients with intact deltoid and those with deltoid compromise with regard to pain, function, range of motion, University of California-Los Angeles (UCLA) shoulder score, or the overall satisfaction with the shoulder. The investigators make the point that all of these patients are still moderately disabled after this surgery and do not have normal shoulder function. However, they emphasize that there was a significant overall improvement in UCLA score postoperatively versus preoperative scores, implying that latissimus dorsi transfer was an effective procedure for salvage after failure of repair of a massive rotator cuff tear.

Warner and Parsons[7] further developed this concept and compared primary latissimus dorsi transfer with transfer as a salvage procedure after failed rotator cuff repair. This study compared outcomes of 16 patients who underwent latissimus dorsi transfer as a salvage procedure for failed rotator cuff repair with those of 6 patients who underwent the transfer as a primary procedure for massive irreparable rotator cuff repair, based on a 7-year experience with this technique. In the 16 revision patients, 3 had undergone more than 1 previous rotator cuff repair and 7 had undergone a distal clavicle resection. Preoperative modified Constant scores were comparable between the groups: mean 37% in the primary group and 36% in the salvage group. At a mean follow-up of 25 months, the relative gain between preoperative and postoperative forward flexion was 60° (range, 30°–90°) for the primary group versus 43° (range, 15°–75°) for the revision group. Six patients in the revision group were limited to 90° of active forward flexion or less, whereas all of the patients in the primary group achieved at least 100° of flexion. Five of those 6 patients in the revision group were noted to have deltoid detachment intraoperatively. The modified Constant score of all 6 patients in the primary group improved by more than 30%, but only 1 patient in the revision group improved to this extent. Poor tendon quality, severe fatty degeneration, and deltoid detachment were predictive of poor outcome. Poor tendon quality and severe fatty degeneration occurred with the same frequency in the primary and revision groups, but deltoid detachment was not seen in the primary group, whereas 7 of the 16 revision patients had deltoid detachment. Unlike in Ianotti's study, differences in outcome between those with an injured deltoid and those with an intact deltoid were statistically significant, both within the revision group and between the revision and primary groups. Rupture of the transferred latissimus dorsi occurred in 1 of 6 primary cases and 7 of 16 revision cases at a mean of 19 months after surgery (range, 3–38 months). The overall incidence was 36%, including a 17% rupture rate for the primary group and a 44% rupture rate for the revision group. Outcomes in the primary group of patients were comparable with those of Gerber's original series; however, outcomes in the revision group suggested that when latissimus dorsi transfer is used as a salvage procedure after failed rotator cuff repair, it results in more limited gains in subjective and objective outcomes. Almost 20% of the revision patients reported a poor outcome. The investigators believed that deltoid deficiency had a profound effect on clinical outcome in revision cases, given that all patients with deltoid deficiency had a failed previous rotator cuff repair. They highlighted the importance of patient selection for latissimus dorsi transfer as a salvage procedure, because concomitant shoulder disease and its effect on shoulder function are a factor in inferior outcomes. The rotator cuff tear configuration did not seem to influence outcomes. The investigators concluded that an intact deltoid is mandatory for restoration of shoulder function. Birmingham and Neviaser[49] also found that deltoid function was linked to the degree of improvement after latissimus dorsi transfer for failed rotator cuff repair.

More recent modifications to the technique of latissimus dorsi transfer include harvesting the tendon along with a small piece of bone, which enabled direct transosseous bone-to-bone healing of the transfer,[50] a single-incision technique,[51,52] and a further modification of the single-incision technique to use a minimally invasive approach only expose the humeral tendon insertion and the site of transfer reinsertion.[53] Although there are theoretic advantages to these modifications, none has given results superior to Gerber's original series. The latissimus dorsi tendon transfer can successfully restore shoulder function but has not been shown to halt progression of cuff tear arthropathy.

Pectoralis Major Transfer

Pectoralis major transfer is an option for the massive anterosuperior rotator cuff tear. Repair of chronic subscapularis ruptures can be challenging, and has not led to favorable results. Young and Rockwood[54] initially reported on transfer of the pectoralis minor for 4 patients and the pectoralis major for 1 patient after failed Bristow procedures, with good or excellent results. Encouraged by these early results for patients without complete detachment of subscapularis, Wirth and Rockwood[55] began in 1980 to perform this transfer for patients with complete absence of subscapularis. They performed pectoralis major or pectoralis minor transfers in 13 shoulders between 1980 and 1994 for irreparable subscapularis tears (defined as complete absence of the subscapularis) in the setting of anterior glenohumeral instability. A satisfactory result was achieved in 10 shoulders according to the Neer and Foster grading system, and an unsatisfactory result in 3 shoulders, at a mean of 5 years postoperatively. All 3 of the shoulders with an unsatisfactory result had undergone at least 2 previous reconstructive operations. These shoulders had persistent pain, poor strength, and anterior laxity. One had a new trauma that precipitated the failure of her tendon transfer. All 10 shoulders with a satisfactory result showed active contraction of the transferred muscle and diminished anterior glenohumeral translation. These patients had slight or no pain with activities of daily living or work.

Resch and colleagues[56] reported on older patients (mean age 65 years) with irreparable subscapularis tears whom they treated with subcoracoid pectoralis major transfer. The superior half to two-thirds of pectoralis major was used as a substitute for the subscapularis tendon in 12 patients. The pectoralis muscle transfer was routed behind the conjoined tendon (coracobrachialis and short head of the biceps) to the lesser tuberosity to adapt the orientation of the pectoralis to that of the subscapularis (**Fig. 8**). At a mean follow-up of 28 months, there were 5 excellent outcomes, 4 good, 3 fair, and no poor outcomes. The mean Constant score improved from 26.9 to 67.1, and ultrasonography showed healing of the transfer in all 12 patients.

Elhassan and colleagues[22] divided their group of 30 patients treated with pectoralis major transfers into 3 distinct subgroups: in group I were 11 patients with a failed instability procedure and a mean age of 37 years; in group II were 8 patients with subscapularis rupture after total arthroplasty or hemiarthroplasty and a mean age of 55 years; and in group III were 11 patients with a massive rotator cuff tear involving subscapularis and a mean age of 58 years. All patients were treated with split transfer of the sternal head of pectoralis major passed under the clavicular head, which allows the clavicular head to act as a fulcrum for the transferred sternal head when it contracts.

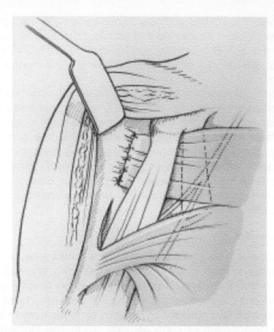

Fig. 8. Schematic view of the course of the transferred pectoralis major under the conjoint tendon. *(Reprinted from* Resch H, Povacz P, Ritter E, et al. Transfer of the pectoralis major muscle for the treatment of irreparable rupture of the subscapularis tendon. JBJS Am 2000;82:375; with permission.)

This strategy also helps guide the axis of pull of the sternal head of the pectoralis major to be more in line with the vector of the subscapularis. The vector of pull of the transferred pectoralis major is still anterior to the chest wall, in contrast to the vector of the subscapularis, which is posterior to the chest wall. This is a feature of all techniques of pectoralis major transfer (direct, subcoracoid deep to conjoint tendon, and deep to clavicular head). At a minimum of 2-year follow-up, pain had improved in 7 of 11 patients in each of group I and group III, but only in 1 of 8 patients in group II. Constant scores improved in all groups, but the improvement was least in the group with subscapularis rupture after shoulder arthroplasty. Failure of the tendon transfer was highest in group II (6 of 8 patients), compared with 3 of 11 in group I and 4 of 11 in group III. The investigators concluded that in patients with irreparable subscapularis tear after shoulder arthroplasty, there is a high risk of failure of transfer of pectoralis major, particularly if there is preoperative anterior subluxation of the humeral head. In patients with isolated subscapularis insufficiency after a failed stabilization procedure, improvement in pain and function can be expected in those who have a concentric glenohumeral joint preoperatively. However, if the shoulder joint is subluxed or not concentric, the transfer of pectoralis tendon is more likely to fail and alternative treatment such as a bone block, transfer of the coracoid, or capsular reconstruction using tendon allograft or autograft should be considered as a salvage procedure.

Biomechanically, routing the transferred pectoralis major tendon under the conjoint tendon is preferred to routing the transfer over the conjoint tendon (**Fig. 9**), but there is no evidence that the technically less demanding technique over the conjoint tendon provides clinically inferior results.[57,58] In a series of 30 patients (average age 53 years) with pectoralis major transfer over the conjoined tendon, the mean relative Constant

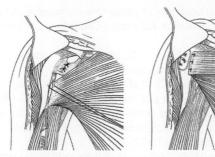

Fig. 9. Schematic view of the course of the transferred pectoralis major over the conjoint tendon. (*Reprinted from* Jost B, Puskas GJ, Lustenberger A, et al. Outcome of pectoralis major transfer for the treatment of irreparable subscapularis tears. J Bone Joint Surg Am 2003;85-A(10):1947; with permission.)

score improved from preoperative 47% to postoperative 70% after a follow-up of 32 months.[58] Whereas patients with an isolated subscapularis tear or an additional repairable supraspinatus tear had a postoperative relative Constant score of 79%, patients with an additional irreparable supraspinatus (and infraspinatus) tear had a clearly inferior clinical outcome, with a mean Constant score of only 49% at final follow-up. Overall, the results were not different compared with patients in whom the transfer was performed under the conjoined tendon.[58]

Deltoid Flap Reconstruction

European surgeons have used a deltoid flap to reconstruct posterosuperior tears, with variable results. Lu and colleagues[59] reported satisfactory medium-term results in terms of pain relief and improvement in shoulder function with this technique; however, long-term outcomes were poor: 50% of the deltoid flaps had ruptured at a mean follow-up of 13.9 years, and 70% of shoulders had stage 2 or 3 osteoarthritis. No predictive factor for deltoid flap rupture was identified. Glanzmann and colleagues[60] reported minor functional gains but acceptable pain relief and patient satisfaction after deltoid flap; however, ultrasonography showed survival of only 16.5% of the deltoid flaps at mid-term and 12.5% at long-term follow-up. In both cases, the investigators do not recommend further use of this procedure.

ACKNOWLEDGMENTS

The authors wish to acknowledge the contribution of Jeffrey D. Tompson, BS, Harvard Shoulder Service Research Assistant, for his assistance in the preparation of this article.

REFERENCES

1. Patte D. Classification of rotator cuff lesions. Clin Orthop Relat Res 1990;(254): 81–6.
2. Cofield RH, Parvizi J, Hoffmeyer PJ, et al. Surgical repair of chronic rotator cuff tears. A prospective long-term study. J Bone Joint Surg Am 2001;83-A(1):71–7.
3. Burkhart SS. Arthroscopic treatment of massive rotator cuff tears. Clinical results and biomechanical rationale. Clin Orthop Relat Res 1991;(267):45–56.

4. Rockwood CA Jr. The management of patients with massive defects in the rotator cuff. Presidential Guest Speaker Address. Orlando (FL): Mid-America Orthopaedic Association; 1986.

5. Gerber C, Fuchs B, Hodler J. The results of repair of massive tears of the rotator cuff. J Bone Joint Surg Am 2000;82(4):505–15.

6. Warner JJ, Endres NK, Higgins LD, et al. Massive irreparable tendon tears of the rotator cuff: salvage options. Instr Course Lect 2008;57:153–66.

7. Warner JJ, Parsons IM. Latissimus dorsi tendon transfer: a comparative analysis of primary and salvage reconstruction of massive, irreparable rotator cuff tears. J Shoulder Elbow Surg 2001;10(6):514–21.

8. Gartsman GM. Arthroscopic acromioplasty for lesions of the rotator cuff. J Bone Joint Surg Am 1990;72(2):169–80.

9. Hawkins RJ, Misamore GW, Hobeika PE. Surgery for full-thickness rotator-cuff tears. J Bone Joint Surg Am 1985;67(9):1349–55.

10. Levy HJ, Gardner RD, Lemak LJ. Arthroscopic subacromial decompression in the treatment of full-thickness rotator cuff tears. Arthroscopy 1991;7(1):8–13.

11. Rockwood CA Jr, Williams GR Jr, Burkhead WZ Jr. Debridement of degenerative, irreparable lesions of the rotator cuff. J Bone Joint Surg Am 1995;77(6):857–66.

12. Burkhart SS, Nottage WM, Ogilvie-Harris DJ, et al. Partial repair of irreparable rotator cuff tears. Arthroscopy 1994;10(4):363–70.

13. Walch G, Edwards TB, Boulahia A, et al. Arthroscopic tenotomy of the long head of the biceps in the treatment of rotator cuff tears: clinical and radiographic results of 307 cases. J Shoulder Elbow Surg 2005;14(3):238–46.

14. Badhe SP, Lawrence TM, Smith FD, et al. An assessment of porcine dermal xenograft as an augmentation graft in the treatment of extensive rotator cuff tears. J Shoulder Elbow Surg 2008;17(Suppl 1):35S–9S.

15. Chaudhury S, Holland C, Thompson MS, et al. Tensile and shear mechanical properties of rotator cuff repair patches. J Shoulder Elbow Surg 2011;21(9):1168–76.

16. Wong I, Burns J, Snyder S. Arthroscopic GraftJacket repair of rotator cuff tears. J Shoulder Elbow Surg 2010;19(Suppl 2):104–9.

17. Boykin RE, Friedman DJ, Zimmer ZR, et al. Suprascapular neuropathy in a shoulder referral practice. J Shoulder Elbow Surg 2011;20(6):983–8.

18. Lafosse L, Tomasi A, Corbett S, et al. Arthroscopic release of suprascapular nerve entrapment at the suprascapular notch: technique and preliminary results. Arthroscopy 2007;23(1):34–42.

19. Costouros JG, Porramatikul M, Lie DT, et al. Reversal of suprascapular neuropathy following arthroscopic repair of massive supraspinatus and infraspinatus rotator cuff tears. Arthroscopy 2007;23(11):1152–61.

20. Mallon WJ, Wilson RJ, Basamania CJ. The association of suprascapular neuropathy with massive rotator cuff tears: a preliminary report. J Shoulder Elbow Surg 2006;15(4):395–8.

21. Gerber C. Latissimus dorsi transfer for the treatment of irreparable tears of the rotator cuff. Clin Orthop Relat Res 1992;(275):152–60.

22. Elhassan B, Ozbaydar M, Massimini D, et al. Transfer of pectoralis major for the treatment of irreparable tears of subscapularis: does it work? J Bone Joint Surg Br 2008;90(8):1059–65.

23. Pedowitz RA, Yamaguchi K, Ahmad CS, et al. American Academy of Orthopaedic Surgeons clinical practice guideline on: optimizing the management of rotator cuff problems. J Bone Joint Surg Am 2012;94(2):163–7.

24. Melillo AS, Savoie FH 3rd, Field LD. Massive rotator cuff tears: debridement versus repair. Orthop Clin North Am 1997;28(1):117–24.

25. Neer CS 2nd. Anterior acromioplasty for the chronic impingement syndrome in the shoulder: a preliminary report. J Bone Joint Surg Am 1972;54(1):41–50.
26. Zvijac JE, Levy HJ, Lemak LJ. Arthroscopic subacromial decompression in the treatment of full thickness rotator cuff tears: a 3- to 6-year follow-up. Arthroscopy 1994;10(5):518–23.
27. Ellman H, Kay SP, Wirth M. Arthroscopic treatment of full-thickness rotator cuff tears: 2- to 7-year follow-up study. Arthroscopy 1993;9(2):195–200.
28. Gartsman GM. Massive, irreparable tears of the rotator cuff. Results of operative debridement and subacromial decompression. J Bone Joint Surg Am 1997;79(5): 715–21.
29. Montgomery TJ, Yerger B, Savoie FH. Management of rotator cuff tears: a comparison of arthroscopic debridement and surgical repair. J Shoulder Elbow Surg 1994;3(2):70–8.
30. Wiley AM. Superior humeral dislocation. A complication following decompression and debridement for rotator cuff tears. Clin Orthop Relat Res 1991;(263):135–41.
31. Fagelman M, Sartori M, Freedman KB, et al. Biomechanics of coracoacromial arch modification. J Shoulder Elbow Surg 2007;16(1):101–6.
32. Flatow EL, Weinstein DM, Duralde XA, et al. Coracoacromial ligament preservation in rotator cuff surgery. J Shoulder Elbow Surg 1993;2(1):S63.
33. Fenlin JM Jr, Chase JM, Rushton SA, et al. Tuberoplasty: creation of an acromio-humeral articulation–a treatment option for massive, irreparable rotator cuff tears. J Shoulder Elbow Surg 2002;11(2):136–42.
34. Burkhart SS. Arthroscopic treatment of massive rotator cuff tears. Clin Orthop Relat Res 2001;(390):107–18.
35. Tauro JC. Arthroscopic "interval slide" in the repair of large rotator cuff tears. Arthroscopy 1999;15(5):527–30.
36. Hsu JE, Reuther KE, Sarver JJ, et al. Restoration of anterior-posterior rotator cuff force balance improves shoulder function in a rat model of chronic massive tears. J Orthop Res 2011;29(7):1028–33.
37. Mazzocca AD, Bollier M, Fehsenfeld D, et al. Biomechanical evaluation of margin convergence. Arthroscopy 2011;27(3):330–8.
38. Boileau P, Baque F, Valerio L, et al. Isolated arthroscopic biceps tenotomy or tenodesis improves symptoms in patients with massive irreparable rotator cuff tears. J Bone Joint Surg Am 2007;89(4):747–57.
39. Warner JP, Krushell RJ, Masquelet A, et al. Anatomy and relationships of the suprascapular nerve: anatomical constraints to mobilization of the supraspinatus and infraspinatus muscles in the management of massive rotator-cuff tears. J Bone Joint Surg Am 1992;74(1):36–45.
40. Vad VB, Southern D, Warren RF, et al. Prevalence of peripheral neurologic injuries in rotator cuff tears with atrophy. J Shoulder Elbow Surg 2003;12(4):333–6.
41. Lafosse L, Piper K, Lanz U. Arthroscopic suprascapular nerve release: indications and technique. J Shoulder Elbow Surg 2011;20(Suppl 2):S9–13.
42. Warner JJ. Management of massive irreparable rotator cuff tears: the role of tendon transfer. Instr Course Lect 2001;50:63–71.
43. Gerber C, Vinh TS, Hertel R, et al. Latissimus dorsi transfer for the treatment of massive tears of the rotator cuff. A preliminary report. Clin Orthop Relat Res 1988;(232):51–61.
44. L'Episcopo JB. Tendon transposition in obstetrical paralysis. Am J Surg 1934; 232:51–61.
45. Gerber C, Maquieira G, Espinosa N. Latissimus dorsi transfer for the treatment of irreparable rotator cuff tears. J Bone Joint Surg Am 2006;88(1):113–20.

46. Morelli M, Nagamori J, Gilbart M, et al. Latissimus dorsi tendon transfer for massive irreparable cuff tears: an anatomic study. J Shoulder Elbow Surg 2008;17(1):139–43.

47. Iannotti JP, Hennigan S, Herzog R, et al. Latissimus dorsi tendon transfer for irreparable posterosuperior rotator cuff tears. Factors affecting outcome. J Bone Joint Surg Am 2006;88(2):342–8.

48. Miniaci A, MacLeod M. Transfer of the latissimus dorsi muscle after failed repair of a massive tear of the rotator cuff. A two to five-year review. J Bone Joint Surg Am 1999;81(8):1120–7.

49. Birmingham PM, Neviaser RJ. Outcome of latissimus dorsi transfer as a salvage procedure for failed rotator cuff repair with loss of elevation. J Shoulder Elbow Surg 2008;17(6):871–4.

50. Moursy M, Forstner R, Koller H, et al. Latissimus dorsi tendon transfer for irreparable rotator cuff tears: a modified technique to improve tendon transfer integrity. J Bone Joint Surg Am 2009;91(8):1924–31.

51. Habermeyer P, Magosch P, Rudolph T, et al. Transfer of the tendon of latissimus dorsi for the treatment of massive tears of the rotator cuff: a new single-incision technique. J Bone Joint Surg Br 2006;88(2):208–12.

52. Gerhardt C, Lehmann L, Lichtenberg S, et al. Modified L'Episcopo tendon transfers for irreparable rotator cuff tears: 5-year follow-up. Clin Orthop Relat Res 2010;468(6):1572–7.

53. Lehmann LJ, Mauerman E, Strube T, et al. Modified minimally invasive latissimus dorsi transfer in the treatment of massive rotator cuff tears: a two-year follow-up of 26 consecutive patients. Int Orthop 2010;34(3):377–83.

54. Young DC, Rockwood CA Jr. Complications of a failed Bristow procedure and their management. J Bone Joint Surg Am 1991;73(7):969–81.

55. Wirth MA, Rockwood CA Jr. Operative treatment of irreparable rupture of the subscapularis. J Bone Joint Surg Am 1997;79(5):722–31.

56. Resch H, Povacz P, Ritter E, et al. Transfer of the pectoralis major muscle for the treatment of irreparable rupture of the subscapularis tendon. J Bone Joint Surg Am 2000;82(3):372–82.

57. Resch H, Povacz P, Ritter E, et al. Pectoralis major muscle transfer for irreparable rupture of the subscapularis and supraspinatus tendon. Tech Shoulder Elbow Surg 2002;3(3):167–73.

58. Jost B, Puskas GJ, Lustenberger A, et al. Outcome of pectoralis major transfer for the treatment of irreparable subscapularis tears. J Bone Joint Surg Am 2003; 85-A(10):1944–51.

59. Lu XW, Verborgt O, Gazielly DF. Long-term outcomes after deltoid muscular flap transfer for irreparable rotator cuff tears. J Shoulder Elbow Surg 2008;17(5): 732–7.

60. Glanzmann MC, Goldhahn J, Flury M, et al. Deltoid flap reconstruction for massive rotator cuff tears: mid- and long-term functional and structural results. J Shoulder Elbow Surg 2010;19(3):439–45.

Reverse Total Shoulder Arthroplasty for Irreparable Rotator Cuff Tears and Cuff Tear Arthropathy

Miguel A. Ramirez, MD, Jose Ramirez, MA, Anand M. Murthi, MD*

KEYWORDS

- Reverse shoulder arthroplasty • Total shoulder replacement • Cuff tear arthropathy
- Irreparable rotator cuff tear • Shoulder pseudoparalysis

KEY POINTS

- Rotator cuff arthropathy is the end-stage result of rotator cuff tears and consists of rotator cuff tear, glenohumeral arthritis, superior humeral migration, and a pseudoparalytic shoulder in a subset of patients.
- Hemiarthroplasty has yielded unpredictable results in patients with rotator cuff arthropathy.
- Reverse shoulder arthroplasty was designed to restore elevation in the cuff-deficient shoulder by increasing the efficiency of the deltoid as the primary elevator of the arm.
- Reverse shoulder arthroplasty can be a reasonable salvage procedure for the irreparable rotator cuff in the older patient.
- Reverse shoulder arthroplasty in cuff tear arthropathy has yielded good outcomes in terms of pain and function scores in the short term. Long-term studies are yet needed to determine the longevity of these devices.

INTRODUCTION

Cuff tear arthropathy and massive, irreparable cuff tears are challenging diagnoses facing orthopedic surgeons. Until recently, hemiarthroplasty was considered the best option in these patients, and although pain scores improved with this procedure, functional scores left much to be desired.[1–3] Reverse shoulder arthroplasty (RSA) was developed in the 1980s as a novel way of treating these pathologies. This article summarizes the biomechanics of reverse shoulder arthroplasty and reviews the available literature for its use in cuff tear arthropathy and irreparable cuff tears.

Department of Orthopaedic Surgery, Union Memorial Hospital, 3333 North Calvert Street, Suite 400, Baltimore, MD 21218, USA
* Corresponding author.
E-mail address: amurthi@gcoa.net

Clin Sports Med 31 (2012) 749–759
http://dx.doi.org/10.1016/j.csm.2012.07.009
0278-5919/12/$ – see front matter © 2012 Elsevier Inc. All rights reserved.

HISTORY OF RSA

Although the first reported shoulder replacement was performed by Dr Jules Émile Péan in 1893, for treatment of tuberculosis,[4,5] it was not until 80 years later that the modern-day shoulder arthroplasty era began with the introduction of the Neer 1 shoulder prosthesis by Neer and Kirby in 1970.[6] This new implant improved pain and function in patients with end-stage arthritis and an intact rotator cuff. There was a high rate of glenoid loosening in patients with rotator cuff arthropathy[7] and, therefore, new designs were developed to prevent glenoid component failure.

RSA was born out of a need to replicate the biomechanics of other weight-bearing joints. Initial highly constrained designs like the Stanmore shoulder and Leeds shoulder[4,8,9] used the action of the deltoid to restore function around a fixed center of rotation. These designs were associated with high rates of clinical failure because of loosening of the glenoid components as a result of large, eccentric forces on the glenoid component with a lateralized center of rotation on the humerus.[7,10] By 1983, total shoulder arthroplasty in those patients had such poor outcomes that Neer and Kirby advocated for hemiarthroplasty with "limited goals" for recovery.[6]

In 1987, Grammont introduced a novel concept for RSA: a redesigned reverse ball and socket prosthesis that created a medialized center of rotation (within the scapula), which allowed the deltoid to achieve restoration of shoulder elevation in patients with cuff tear arthropathy.[11] Grammont's early work in 1993 helped revitalize interest in RSA and laid the foundation for modern designs.[12] The Delta 3 prosthesis (DePuy, Warsaw, IN) become the prototype for modern RSA designs (**Fig. 1**).[11]

BIOMECHANICS OF RSA

Paul Grammont's vision of the reverse total shoulder system arose from his extensive study of human evolution.[13] In his studies, Grammont observed that upright posture in humans led to an evolutionary relative attrition of the supraspinatus muscle compared with the deltoid. As a result, the acromion became more lateralized, effectively increasing the deltoid's abduction component. Understanding this, Grammont conceived that he could overcome rotator cuff weakness by lateralizing the acromion and medializing the joint center of rotation.[13,14] In a deltoid simulator, Grammont was able to show that a 10-mm medial displacement of the center of rotation increases the abduction moment of the middle deltoid by 20% at 60° of elevation. A 10-mm inferior displacement of the center of rotation increases deltoid abduction moment by 30% at 60° of elevation.[11,12,14]

The Delta III reverse shoulder prosthesis developed by Grammont transferred the center of rotation medially and lengthened the humerus, essentially turning the deltoid into a more efficient elevator of the arm and increasing glenohumeral compression, which stabilizes the prosthetic articulation. The Delta III reverse shoulder system is composed of a humeral stem, humeral neck, polyethylene cup, glenosphere, and glenoid baseplate. This novel design differs from previous reverse shoulder systems in that a large, neckless ball is placed on the glenoid side and a small cup set at an inclination of 155° is placed on the humeral side (see **Fig. 1**). This design allows for a fixed, medialized center of rotation, which reduces torque on the glenoid, thereby decreasing the incidence of glenoid loosening seen in previous designs. The design increases acromiohumeral distance, restoring deltoid tension and stabilizing the articulation (**Fig. 2**).[11,15] Moreover, placing the center of rotation at the scapula recruits a larger proportion of the anterior and posterior deltoid, thus rendering it a more efficient and more powerful elevator of the arm.

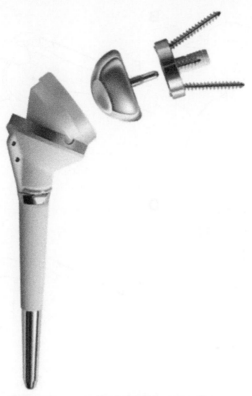

Fig. 1. The delta 3 prosthesis. (*Reprinted from* Boileau P, Watkinson DJ, Hatzidakis AM, et al. Grammont reverse prosthesis: design, rationale, and biomechanics. J Shoulder Elbow Surg 2005;14(Suppl 1):147S–61S; with permission from Elsevier.)

Use of the Delta III reverse prosthesis requires careful patient selection. Scapular notching, defined as humero-glenoid impingement leading to lysis, has been reported with this prosthesis in 44% to 96% of cases.[16] Also, although the deltoid is a powerful abductor and elevator of the arm, it is a weak external rotator. Patients with cuff arthropathy often have a deficient posterior cuff, including teres minor, and therefore often require muscle transfers to regain external rotation strength.[16,17] Medialization of the humerus may result in a loss of the normal deltoid contour, which may be cosmetically unappealing, especially in thin female patients. The arm is often longer with lengthening of the humerus. All of these factors should be carefully discussed with the patient preoperatively because of their potential affect on postoperative satisfaction.

RSA FOR IRREPARABLE CUFF TEARS WITHOUT ARTHRITIS

Massive rotator cuff tears can result in a change in shoulder biomechanics by creating a muscle force imbalance. In the shoulder with an intact rotator cuff, the cuff serves as a fulcrum that translates the shear force of the deltoid into a rotating force, resulting in shoulder elevation.[11] This effect is lost in shoulders with massive cuff tears, leading to proximal migration of the humeral head and loss of shoulder elevation.[11] This entity has been described as pseudoparalysis of the shoulder.[17]

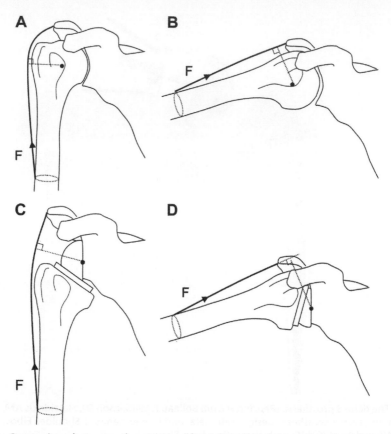

Fig. 2. Comparison between the centers of rotation between native shoulder and RSA. Center of rotation is depicted with arm at the side (*A*), at abduction (*B*), and after RSA (*C, D*). F, force. Medialization of the center of rotation lengthens the lever arm of the deltoid, rendering it a more powerful elevator of the arm. Copyright 2009 American Academy of Orthopedic Surgeons. (*From* Gerber C, Pennington SD, Nyffeler RW. Reverse total shoulder arthroplasty. J Am Acad Orthop Surg 2009;17(5):284–9; with permission. © 2009 American Academy of Orthopaedic Surgeons.)

Repairing the rotator cuff can restore the shoulder biomechanics as well as provide pain relief; however, rotator cuff repair may not be possible because of tendon loss, poor tissue for repair, or muscular fatty atrophy. In this setting, the shoulder surgeon is faced with the task of treating a muscular imbalance with a prosthetic device.

The use of RSA for irreparable cuff tears without arthritis is an extension of the indications for RSA, and, as such, should be considered carefully. Individual patient symptoms, age, and functional demands must be critically evaluated. In our practice, RSA in these patients is strictly a salvage operation in which other modalities have failed. The ideal candidate is the older patient with low functional demand who has failed nonoperative treatment and/or rotator cuff repair and continues to have significant pain and dysfunction.

With careful patient selection, RSA outcomes have been good in patients with irreparable cuff tears. In a Swiss study by Werner and colleagues,[18] the investigators studied RSA in 58 patients with irreparable cuff tears and active elevation less than 90°. The investigators found that the relative constant score improved from 29% to

64%, and elevation increased from 42 to 100°. Total complication rate for all-comers was 50%, including all minor complications. The overall reoperation rate was 33%. The investigators concluded that RSA is a reasonable salvage operation for patients with irreparable cuff tears.

A more recent study by Wall and colleagues,[10] looking at RSA for different etiologies at an average of 39.9 months, found that RSA in massive irreparable cuff tears was able to significantly improve constant scores from 28 to 63 points and to increase average elevation from 94° to 143°.

Mulieri and colleagues[19] performed reverse shoulder arthroplasty in 72 shoulders with massive cuff tears and preoperative elevation less than 90° and followed them for an average of 53 months. They observed an improvement of American Shoulder and Elbow Surgeons scores from 33.3 to 75.4. Patients also saw improvement in active elevation from 54° to 134°, abduction from 49° to 125°, and internal rotation from S1 to L2. There were 12 complications (20%) and an implant survival of 90.7% at 53 months. The investigators also concluded that RSA is a reasonable salvage option in patients with massive cuff tears without arthritis, at least in the short term.

Although results of RSA in massive irreparable cuff tears seems promising, it cannot be overemphasized that careful patient selection is critical to postoperative success. A clear contraindication to RSA is deltoid dysfunction, because the deltoid is the prime elevator of the arm in RSA.[20,21] Care should be taken to evaluate deltoid competency preoperatively, especially in the patients with traumatic cuff tear who can have a superimposed axillary nerve palsy.

A relative contraindication to RSA is good active range of motion despite rotator cuff tear, as RSA offers little if any benefit to this population. In these patients, our standard treatment is nonoperative care with physical therapy and/or injections to manage symptoms. Shoulder arthroscopy and debridement with biceps tenotomy/tenodesis may also provide pain relief in patients refractory to injections and physical therapy. Care to maintain the integrity of the coracoacromial arch is crucial to maintain function in these patients.

RSA FOR CUFF TEAR ARTHROPATHY
Pathophysiology of Cuff Tear Arthropathy

The first description of cuff tear arthropathy (CTA) was by Charles Neer in 1981, when he described a process of massive rotator cuff tear associated with proximal migration of the humerus, acetabularization of the acromion, femoralization of the humerus, and glenohumeral erosion.[2,22] Neer proposed 2 mechanisms leading to cuff arthropathy: mechanical and nutritional. The mechanical hypothesis suggested that a massive cuff tear leads to either recurrent instability or superior migration of the humeral head with abnormal wear of the acromion, acromioclavicular joint, and coracoid. The nutritional hypothesis stated that a massive cuff tear leads to reduced motion and loss of "water-tight" joint space. The cumulative effect of this is disuse osteoporosis, biomechanical changes in glycosaminoglycan content leading to cartilage atrophy, and the subchondral collapse seen in CTA. All of these mechanisms result in abnormal trauma leading to cuff arthropathy.[2,22]

Halverson and colleagues[23] introduced an entity that they termed the "Milwaukee shoulder." This condition was characterized by hydroxyapatite deposition in the glenohumeral joint, with an interleukin-1 proliferative synovitis that potentiates collagenase and protease activity resulting in joint destruction in patients with massive cuff tears.[24] Collins and Harryman[25] subsequently postulated a unifying hypothesis of CTA in which superior migration of the humeral head and instability of the coracoacromial arch sets off an abnormal inflammatory cascade leading to crystal deposition and joint destruction.

Hemiarthroplasty for CTA

Given the poor results of total shoulder replacement in patients with CTA, Neer and colleagues[2] advocated shoulder hemiarthroplasty as a more reliable treatment for CTA. They proposed "limited goals" criteria as a benchmark to judge success in treatment of cuff arthropathy.[6] Neer believed that goals of treatment should prioritize pain relief above return of function.

Using Neer's "limited goals" criteria as their end point, several studies have found success in treating cuff tear arthropathy with hemiarthroplasty. In a study by Williams and Rockwood,[26] 21 patients received hemiarthroplasty for CTA. Although pain was improved in 18 of 21 patients, active elevation was only 120°. Other studies have seen similar results in terms of pain relief, but even less postoperative function. Sanchez-Sotelo and colleagues[27] reported 73% pain relief, but only 91° of active elevation, which deteriorated over time with worsening elevation and superior glenoid erosion.

More recently, Goldberg and colleagues[28] investigated long-term outcomes of hemiarthroplasty for CTA. Of their 34 patients, 25 had an average follow-up of 10 years. Twenty-five (73%) of 34 met Neer's limited goals criteria for a satisfactory outcome. Mean active elevation improved from 78° to 111° and active external rotation improved from 15° to 38°. The investigators concluded that hemiarthroplasty provides good long-term results in patients with CTA and no pseudoparalysis on physical examination.

Reverse Total Shoulder for Cuff Arthropathy

RSA was developed as an attractive treatment modality for patients with CTA. The goals of this device are to go beyond Neer's limited goals criteria by providing pain relief and improving postoperative function.

Grammont and colleagues[14] performed the first study of RSA in CTA in 1996. In this study, 16 patients received the Grammont Delta III prosthesis and were followed for an average of 27 months. At follow-up, average constant scores improved from 14 to 69. There was a reoperation rate of 13%. In a 1997 study, of 71 patients with cuff tear arthropathy, De Buttet and colleagues[29] found that patients had a mean postoperative elevation of 120° at an average of 24 months. Reoperation rate in these patients was 4.2%.

More recently, Boileau and colleagues[30] received the Neer award for their study on RSA for various indications. In their series, 45 patients received the Grammont Delta III prosthesis (DePuy, Warsaw, IN), including 21 patients with primary CTA, 5 with fracture, and 19 with revision after failed previous operative intervention. Patients were followed prospectively for an average of 40 months. Average elevation improved from 53° to 123°, external rotation from 9° to 14°, and internal rotation from S1 to L3. Constant scores improved from 18 to 66 ($P<.001$). The authors reported 14 complications in 11 patients. Nine of these complications occurred in the revision group. Some of the complications included axillary nerve palsy, hematoma, 3 dislocations, intraoperative glenoid fracture, 3 deep infection, and a periprosthetic fracture. Of the 21 patients with primary RSA for CTA, none required a revision surgery. The investigators concluded that RSA improved pain and forward elevation in patients with CTA, with a low complication rate at short-term follow-up (5% at 49 months). Revision surgery carried a much higher complication rate of 45%.

In the largest series to date, Sirveaux and colleagues[31] performed a multicenter review of 80 patients who received the Grammont Delta reverse prosthesis at a mean follow-up of 44 months. At final follow-up, 96% of patients had minimal or no pain. Patients in this cohort saw an average improvement in active forward elevation from 73° to 138°. Active external rotation at 90° improved from 17° to 40°. There was no difference in active internal rotation or external rotation at 0° of abduction. Overall, 96% of patients had minimal or no pain at follow-up; however, during this 44-month period of follow-up, there were 5 cases of glenoid loosening, dissociation of glenoid component in 7, device failure in 3, scapular notching in 49, and deep infection in 1 needing revision. The investigators concluded that RSA is a reasonable treatment for CTA with promising short-term results.

To our knowledge, there are no published randomized studies comparing hemiarthroplasty to RSA in cuff arthropathy. Given the review of the available literature, we believe that RSA is a better option in terms of regaining function in patients with CTA. In fact, a recent study by Coe and colleagues[1] suggests that RSA may be more cost-effective than hemiarthroplasty for CTA when utility gained from the operation, utility lost from complications, and costs of the prosthesis are factored. We also feel it is important to stress that RSA studies have mostly been short-term studies and that long-term efficacy of this treatment is still unknown. Longer follow-up of the current existing series is necessary to make recommendations regarding the long-term outcomes of these devices.

Complications

RSA represents a method to "salvage" a shoulder that has severe functional and anatomic impairment that, in some cases, have proven to be refractory to surgical treatment. However, complications have been reported in up to 50% of cases in some series.[18] Common complications include prosthetic dislocation, implant loosening, infection, scapular notching, acromial stress fractures, deltoid detachment, and deterioration of function over time, among others.[32,33]

Infection

The rate of infection in primary cases of RSA has been reported from to be 1% to 10%.[10,18,33,34] These rates tend to be higher compared with the reported rates of 0.7% to 2.2% in total shoulder arthroplasty.[35,36] The increased risk of infection in RSA may because of the prosthetic design. It is believed that the reverse orientation of the prosthesis forms a large subacromial dead space where hematomas may form.[15] Infections are most likely to develop as short-term postoperative complications and can be treated with lavage, debridement, polyethylene exchange, and antibiotics. Those infections that develop after 3 months are typically less responsive to debridement and may require prosthesis revision, with parenteral antibiotics and a period of shoulder antibiotic spacer placement.[34]

Reoperation

Wall and colleagues[10] reported the need for revision or prosthesis removal in 3.5% (8 of 227) of patients treated with RSA for various etiologies at an average of 39.9 months postoperatively. In that series, radiographic evidence of glenoid loosening was seen in 2 of 227 patients. These patients were subsequently treated with hemiarthroplasty, which achieved pain relief but little improvement in shoulder function. The investigators attributed loosening to surgical error. Hemiarthroplasty, however, is contraindicated in those patients with an incompetent coracoacromial arch because anterosuperior escape may result with extremely poor function and pain.

Werner and colleagues[18] reported higher reoperation rates among patients undergoing primary RSA with Delta III prosthesis for painful pseudoparalysis caused by irreparable rotator cuff dysfunction, 3 (18%) of 17 needing reoperation. The investigators also reported high degrees of patient satisfaction in spite of complications requiring reoperation and found no significant difference in occurrence of complication, subjective shoulder value, Constant score, and patient satisfaction between primary and revision RSA. Patients with a surgical history had a significantly higher rate of reoperation after RSA.

Some investigators suggest, anecdotally, that the 3 complications of hematoma formation requiring evacuation, insufficient deltoid tension causing instability and requiring liner exchange, and infection requiring removal of the prosthesis are the most common reasons for revision in RSA.[15] Furthermore, overall satisfaction with RSA is not influenced by complications requiring revision surgery.[18]

Glenoid loosening

Reliable bony fixation of the glenoid component is crucial to the success of RSA. Unfortunately, failure of the glenoid component in RSA has been reported widely. One large multicenter study on Grammont implants found failures in the glenoid component, which were frequently associated with intraoperative glenoid fracture, screw breakage, and glenoid unscrewing.[29] Postoperative loosing on the glenoid component has been observed in 4.1% of implanted traditional implants with medialized center of rotation followed for more than 2 years.[34] Wall and colleagues[10] reported glenoid loosening in only 2 of 227 patients treated with a Grammont-style prosthesis with medialized center of rotation in RSA for various etiologies. Loosening was attributed to surgical error.

A prospective study of 94 patients who underwent modified RSA with use of 5.0-mm peripheral locking screws for baseplate fixation and a lateralized center of rotation and inferior tilt to the glenosphere reported no mechanical failure of the baseplate at 2-year follow-up, presumably because of reduced micromotion at the baseplate bone interface,[37] a phenomenon that has been previously demonstrated in a biomechanical study.[38] Another biomechanical study[39] also showed the least amount of tensile force and most uniform compressive forces when the glenosphere was tilted 15° inferiorly.[38]

Dislocation

Because the reverse shoulder system is an unconstrained prosthesis, there is concern for stability of the implant. Instability is the most common complication of RSA.[33] Deltoid tension is the primary stabilizer of the prosthesis,[11] and attention should be paid to achieving adequate deltoid tension intraoperatively to prevent future dislocation.[5] Even with meticulous technique, however, dislocation does occur. In previous studies, dislocation rates of 0% to 30% have been reported.[18,40,41] Instability is usually lateral and typically occurs with shoulder extension.

Risk factors for dislocation include deltopectoral approach (compared with superolateral approach), small glenoid size, and poor subscapularis quality.[15] Prevention of shoulder dislocation is predicated on paying meticulous attention to the soft tissue envelope surrounding the prosthesis by increasing the amount of glenosphere offset or augmenting the liner. Often the larger glenosphere will provide greater stability and prevent bony impingement both inferiorly and posteriorly.

Treatment of shoulder dislocations is usually via closed reduction followed by a short interval of sling immobilization (4–6 weeks). If the patient remains unstable, surgical technique must be evaluated and component revision may be necessary. Often an inadequate inferior and posterior capsular release contributes to soft tissue impingement and instability.

Scapular notching

Scapular notching is radiographic evidence of erosion or wear of the lateral pillar of the scapula directly inferior to the glenoid baseplate. This is caused by impingement of the humerus or humeral component onto the glenoid. In Grammont-style prostheses with a medialized center of rotation, scapular notching rates are reported in between 51% and 96% of patients.[30,33] In lateralized glenosphere designs, notching can range from 0% to 13%.[33,40]

Sirveaux and colleagues[31] classified scapular notching into 4 grades. Grade 1 defects are confined to the pillar, Grade 2 extends to the lower screw, Grade 3 surrounds the screw, and Grade 4 defects extend under the baseplate. Grade 4 changes suggest glenoid loosening.

Although this entity is widely reported, the clinical relevance remains uncertain.[32,33] A recent study by Cazeneuve and Cristofari[42] suggests that scapular notching may be correlated with early glenoid loosening and deterioration of Constant scores. In their study, with a mean follow-up of 6 years, the investigators found a notching rate of 63%. These were associated with lower Constant scores; however, only 1 patient had aseptic loosening of the glenoid at follow-up of 12 years.

In a 2011 study, Sadoghi and colleagues[43] found at 42 months that there was no correlation between Constant scores and scapular notching. At 60 months, however, the investigators found that there was a positive correlation between scapular notching and Constant scores as well as range of motion. There was no correlation between notching and implant stability.

Based on the available literature, the effect of scapular notching remains debated given the lack of long-term studies. It is our practice to avoid superior placement of the glenosphere and tilt the glenosphere 10 to 15° inferiorly. Although scapular notching is a radiographic finding, it most probably relates to polyethylene liner wear and third-body debris leading to glenoid lytic changes.

SUMMARY

Based on the available literature, we believe that reverse shoulder arthroplasty is a reasonable treatment modality in patients with CTA and massive irreparable cuff tears. RSA has been shown to increase patient function and decrease pain. There are still a high number of complications related to this procedure; however, with stringent patient selection criteria and meticulous technique, high patient satisfaction scores are typically achieved in these patients, at least in the short term. Further studies are required to evaluate the efficacy these devices in the long term.

REFERENCES

1. Coe MP, Greiwe RM, Joshi R, et al. The cost-effectiveness of reverse total shoulder arthroplasty compared with hemiarthroplasty for rotator cuff tear arthropathy. J Shoulder Elbow Surg 2012. http://dx.doi.org/10.1016/j.jse.2011.10.010.
2. Neer CS 2nd, Craig EV, Fukuda H. Cuff-tear arthropathy. J Bone Joint Surg Am 1983;65(9):1232–44.
3. Zuckerman JD, Scott AJ, Gallagher MA. Hemiarthroplasty for cuff tear arthropathy. J Shoulder Elbow Surg 2000;9(3):169–72.
4. Jazayeri R, Kwon YW. Evolution of the reverse total shoulder prosthesis. Bull NYU Hosp Jt Dis 2011;69(1):50–5.

5. Lugli T. Artificial shoulder joint by Pean (1893): the facts of an exceptional intervention and the prosthetic method. Clin Orthop Relat Res 1978;133:215–8.

6. Neer CS 2nd, Kirby RM. Revision of humeral head and total shoulder arthroplasties. Clin Orthop Relat Res 1982;170:189–95.

7. Franklin JL, Barrett WP, Jackins SE, et al. Glenoid loosening in total shoulder arthroplasty. Association with rotator cuff deficiency. J Arthroplasty 1988;3(1):39–46.

8. Coughlin MJ, Morris JM, West WF. The semiconstrained total shoulder arthroplasty. J Bone Joint Surg Am 1979;61(4):574–81.

9. Kolbel R, Friedebold G. Shoulder joint replacement. Arch Orthop Unfallchir 1973; 76(1):31–9.

10. Wall B, Nove-Josserand L, O'Connor DP, et al. Reverse total shoulder arthroplasty: a review of results according to etiology. J Bone Joint Surg Am 2007; 89(7):1476–85.

11. Grammont P, Trouilloud P, Laffay JP, Deries X. Concept study and realization of a new total shoulder prosthesis [French]. Rhumatologie 1987;39:407–18.

12. Grammont PM, Baulot E. Delta shoulder prosthesis for rotator cuff rupture. Orthopedics 1993;16(1):65–8.

13. Baulot E, Sirveaux F, Boileau P. Grammont's idea: the story of Paul Grammont's functional surgery concept and the development of the reverse principle. Clin Orthop Relat Res 2011;469(9):2425–31.

14. Grammont PM, Baulot E, Chabernaud D. Resultats des 16 premiers cas d'arthroplastie totatale d'epaule le inversee sans ciment pour des omarthroses avec grande rupture de coiffe. Rev Chir Orthop Reparatrice Appar Mot 1996;82(Suppl I):169.

15. Gerber C, Pennington SD, Nyffeler RW. Reverse total shoulder arthroplasty. J Am Acad Orthop Surg 2009;17(5):284–95.

16. Walker M, Brooks J, Willis M, et al. How reverse shoulder arthroplasty works. Clin Orthop Relat Res 2011;469(9):2440–51.

17. Boileau P, Chuinard C, Roussanne Y, et al. Modified latissimus dorsi and teres major transfer through a single delto-pectoral approach for external rotation deficit of the shoulder: as an isolated procedure or with a reverse arthroplasty. J Shoulder Elbow Surg 2007;16(6):671–82.

18. Werner CM, Steinmann PA, Gilbart M, et al. Treatment of painful pseudoparesis due to irreparable rotator cuff dysfunction with the delta III reverse-ball-and-socket total shoulder prosthesis. J Bone Joint Surg Am 2005;87(7):1476–8.

19. Mulieri P, Dunning P, Klein S, et al. Reverse shoulder arthroplasty for the treatment of irreparable rotator cuff tear without glenohumeral arthritis. J Bone Joint Surg Am 2010;92(15):2544–56.

20. Drake GN, O'Connor DP, Edwards TB. Indications for reverse total shoulder arthroplasty in rotator cuff disease. Clin Orthop Relat Res 2010;468(6):1526–33.

21. Feeley BT, Gallo RA, Craig EV. Cuff tear arthropathy: current trends in diagnosis and surgical management. J Shoulder Elbow Surg 2009;18(3):484–9.

22. Macaulay AA, Greiwe RM, Bigliani LU. Rotator cuff deficient arthritis of the glenohumeral joint. Clin Orthop Surg 2010;2(4):196–202.

23. Halverson PB, Cheung HS, McCarty DJ, et al. "Milwaukee shoulder"—association of microspheroids containing hydroxyapatite crystals, active collagenase, and neutral protease with rotator cuff defects. II. Synovial fluid studies. Arthritis Rheum 1981;24(3):474–83.

24. Halverson PB. Crystal deposition disease of the shoulder (including calcific tendonitis and Milwaukee shoulder syndrome). Curr Rheumatol Rep 2003;5(3):244–7.

25. Collins DN, Harryman DT 2nd. Arthroplasty for arthritis and rotator cuff deficiency. Orthop Clin North Am 1997;28(2):225–39.

26. Williams GR Jr, Rockwood CA Jr. Hemiarthroplasty in rotator cuff-deficient shoulders. J Shoulder Elbow Surg 1996;5(5):362–7.
27. Sanchez-Sotelo J, Cofield RH, Rowland CM. Shoulder hemiarthroplasty for glenohumeral arthritis associated with severe rotator cuff deficiency. J Bone Joint Surg Am 2001;83-A(12):1814–22.
28. Goldberg SS, Bell JE, Kim HJ, et al. Hemiarthroplasty for the rotator cuff-deficient shoulder. J Bone Joint Surg Am 2008;90(3):554–9.
29. De Buttet A, Bouchon Y, Capon D, et al. Grammont shoulder arthroplasty for osteoarthritis with massive rotator cuff tears—report of 71 cases. J Shoulder Elbow Surg 1997;6:197 [abstract].
30. Boileau P, Watkinson D, Hatzidakis AM, et al. Neer award 2005: the Grammont reverse shoulder prosthesis: results in cuff tear arthritis, fracture sequelae, and revision arthroplasty. J Shoulder Elbow Surg 2006;15(5):527–40.
31. Sirveaux F, Favard L, Oudet D, et al. Grammont inverted total shoulder arthroplasty in the treatment of glenohumeral osteoarthritis with massive rupture of the cuff. Results of a multicentre study of 80 shoulders. J Bone Joint Surg Br 2004;86(3):388–95.
32. Farshad M, Gerber C. Reverse total shoulder arthroplasty—from the most to the least common complication. Int Orthop 2010;34(8):1075–82.
33. Cheung E, Willis M, Walker M, et al. Complications in reverse total shoulder arthroplasty. J Am Acad Orthop Surg 2011;19(7):439–49.
34. Mole D, Favard L. Excentered scapulohumeral osteoarthritis. Rev Chir Orthop Reparatrice Appar Mot 2007;93(Suppl 6):37–94.
35. Bohsali KI, Wirth MA, Rockwood CA Jr. Complications of total shoulder arthroplasty. J Bone Joint Surg Am 2006;88(10):2279–92.
36. Jahoda D, Pokorny D, Nyc O, et al. Infectious complications of total shoulder arthroplasty. Acta Chir Orthop Traumatol Cech 2008;75(6):422–8.
37. Cuff D, Pupello D, Virani N, et al. Reverse shoulder arthroplasty for the treatment of rotator cuff deficiency. J Bone Joint Surg Am 2008;90(6):1244–51.
38. Harman M, Frankle M, Vasey M, et al. Initial glenoid component fixation in "reverse" total shoulder arthroplasty: a biomechanical evaluation. J Shoulder Elbow Surg 2005;14(1 Suppl S):162S–7S.
39. Gutierrez S, Walker M, Willis M, et al. Effects of tilt and glenosphere eccentricity on baseplate/bone interface forces in a computational model, validated by a mechanical model, of reverse shoulder arthroplasty. J Shoulder Elbow Surg 2011;20(5):732–9.
40. Frankle M, Siegal S, Pupello D, et al. The reverse shoulder prosthesis for glenohumeral arthritis associated with severe rotator cuff deficiency. A minimum two-year follow-up study of sixty patients. J Bone Joint Surg Am 2005;87(8):1697–705.
41. De Wilde L, Sys G, Julien Y, et al. The reversed delta shoulder prosthesis in reconstruction of the proximal humerus after tumour resection. Acta Orthop Belg 2003;69(6):495–500.
42. Cazeneuve JF, Cristofari DJ. The reverse shoulder prosthesis in the treatment of fractures of the proximal humerus in the elderly. J Bone Joint Surg Br 2010;92(4):535–9.
43. Sadoghi P, Leithner A, Vavken P, et al. Infraglenoidal scapular notching in reverse total shoulder replacement: a prospective series of 60 cases and systematic review of the literature. BMC Musculoskelet Disord 2011;19(12):101.

Index

Clin Sports Med 31 (2012) 761–766
http://dx.doi.org/10.1016/S0278-5919(12)00078-6
0278-5919/12/$ – see front matter © 2012 Elsevier Inc. All rights reserved.

sportsmed.theclinics.com

United States Postal Service

Statement of Ownership, Management, and Circulation
(All Periodicals Publications Except Requestor Publications)

1. Publication Title
Clinics in Sports Medicine

2. Publication Number
0 0 0 - 7 0 2

3. Filing Date
9/14/12

4. Issue Frequency
Jan, Apr, Jul, Oct

5. Number of Issues Published Annually
4

6. Annual Subscription Price
$324.00

7. Complete Mailing Address of Known Office of Publication (Not printer) (Street, city, county, state, and ZIP+4®)

Elsevier Inc.
360 Park Avenue South
New York, NY 10010-1710

Contact Person
Stephen Bushing

Telephone (Include area code)
215-239-3688

8. Complete Mailing Address of Headquarters or General Business Office of Publisher (Not printer)

Elsevier Inc., 360 Park Avenue South, New York, NY 10010-1710

9. Full Names and Complete Mailing Addresses of Publisher, Editor, and Managing Editor (Do not leave blank)

Publisher (Name and complete mailing address)

Kim Murphy, Elsevier, Inc., 1600 John F. Kennedy Blvd. Suite 1800, Philadelphia, PA 19103-2899

Editor (Name and complete mailing address)

David Parsons, Elsevier, Inc., 1600 John F. Kennedy Blvd. Suite 1800, Philadelphia, PA 19103-2899

Managing Editor (Name and complete mailing address)

Barbara Cohen-Kligerman, Elsevier, Inc., 1600 John F. Kennedy Blvd. Suite 1800, Philadelphia, PA 19103-2899

10. Owner (Do not leave blank. If the publication is owned by a corporation, give the name and address of the corporation immediately followed by the names and addresses of all stockholders owning or holding 1 percent or more of the total amount of stock. If not owned by a corporation, give the names and addresses of the individual owners. If owned by a partnership or other unincorporated firm, give its name and address as well as those of each individual owner. If the publication is published by a nonprofit organization, give its name and address.)

Full Name	Complete Mailing Address
Wholly owned subsidiary of	1600 John F. Kennedy Blvd., Ste. 1800
Reed/Elsevier, US holdings	Philadelphia, PA 19103-2899

11. Known Bondholders, Mortgagees, and Other Security Holders Owning or Holding 1 Percent or More of Total Amount of Bonds, Mortgages, or Other Securities. If none, check box. ☐ None

Full Name	Complete Mailing Address
N/A	

12. Tax Status (For completion by nonprofit organizations authorized to mail at nonprofit rates) (Check one)
The purpose, function, and nonprofit status of this organization and the exempt status for federal income tax purposes:
☐ Has Not Changed During Preceding 12 Months
☐ Has Changed During Preceding 12 Months (Publisher must submit explanation of change with this statement)

PS Form 3526, September 2007 (Page 1 of 3 (Instructions Page 3)) PSN 7530-01-000-9931 PRIVACY NOTICE: See our Privacy policy in www.usps.com

---

13. Publication Title
Clinics in Sports Medicine

14. Issue Date for Circulation Data Below
July 2012

15. Extent and Nature of Circulation

		Average No. Copies Each Issue During Preceding 12 Months	No. Copies of Single Issue Published Nearest to Filing Date
a. Total Number of Copies (Net press run)		883	830
b. Paid Circulation (By Mail and Outside the Mail)	(1) Mailed Outside-County Paid Subscriptions Stated on PS Form 3541. (Include paid distribution above nominal rate, advertiser's proof copies, and exchange copies)	562	521
	(2) Mailed In-County Paid Subscriptions Stated on PS Form 3541 (Include paid distribution above nominal rate, advertiser's proof copies, and exchange copies)		
	(3) Paid Distribution Outside the Mails Including Sales Through Dealers and Carriers, Street Vendors, Counter Sales, and Other Paid Distribution Outside USPS®	105	110
	(4) Paid Distribution by Other Classes Mailed Through the USPS (e.g. First-Class Mail®)		
c. Total Paid Distribution (Sum of 15b (1), (2), (3), and (4))	▶	667	631
d. Free or Nominal Rate Distribution (By Mail and Outside the Mail)	(1) Free or Nominal Rate Outside-County Copies Included on PS Form 3541	63	65
	(2) Free or Nominal Rate In-County Copies Included on PS Form 3541		
	(3) Free or Nominal Rate Copies Mailed at Other Classes Through the USPS (e.g. First-Class Mail)		
	(4) Free or Nominal Rate Distribution Outside the Mail (Carriers or other means)		
e. Total Free or Nominal Rate Distribution (Sum of 15d (1), (2), (3) and (4))	▶	63	65
f. Total Distribution (Sum of 15c and 15e)	▶	730	696
g. Copies not Distributed (See instructions to publishers #4 (page #3))	▶	153	134
h. Total (Sum of 15f and g)	▶	883	830
i. Percent Paid (15c divided by 15f times 100)	▶	91.37%	90.66%

16. Publication of Statement of Ownership
If the publication is a general publication, publication of this statement is required. Will be printed in the **October 2012** issue of this publication. ☐ Publication not required.

17. Signature and Title of Editor, Publisher, Business Manager, or Owner

Stephen R. Bushing – Inventory/Distribution Coordinator

Date
September 14, 2012

I certify that all information furnished on this form is true and complete. I understand that anyone who furnishes false or misleading information on this form or who omits material or information requested on the form may be subject to criminal sanctions (including fines and imprisonment) and/or civil sanctions (including civil penalties).

PS Form 3526, September 2007 (Page 2 of 3)

Printed and bound by CPI Group (UK) Ltd, Croydon, CR0 4YY

03/10/2024

01040441-0016